D1481732

THE SICK CITADEL

RA
981
A2L48
1983

The Sick Citadel

The American Academic Medical Center and the Public Interest

Irving J. Lewis

*Albert Einstein College of Medicine,
Yeshiva University*

Cecil G. Sheps, M.D.

University of North Carolina at Chapel Hill

 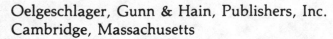 Oelgeschlager, Gunn & Hain, Publishers, Inc.
Cambridge, Massachusetts

Copyright© 1983 by Oelgeschlager, Gunn & Hain, Publishers, Inc. All rights reserved. No part of this publication may be reproduced or transmitted in any form or by any means, electronic or mechanical, including photocopying and recording, or by any information storage or retrieval system, without the prior written consent of the publisher.

International Standard Book Number: 0-89946-173-5

Library of Congress Catalog Card Number: 82-22448

Printed in the U.S.A.

Library of Congress Cataloging in Publication Data

Lewis, Irving J.
  The sick citadel.

  Includes bibliographical references and index.
  1. Medical centers—United States. 2. Medical care—United States. 3. Medical policy—United States. I. Sheps, Cecil G. (Cecil George), 1913- II. Title. [DNLM: 1. Academic medical centers—United States. 2. Health policy—United States. WX 27 L67s]
RA981.A2L48 1982   362.1'0973   82-22448
ISBN 0-89946-173-5

Contents

v

List of Tables

Foreword

Philip R. Lee, M.D.

Professor of Social Medicine
Director, Institute for Health Policy Studies
University of California, San Francisco

The 1980s have brought renewed debate about the major issues in health policy. Equity of access and the containment of health care costs continue to be pivotal issues in that debate. An additional question centers around the role of the private sector, particularly competition and the marketplace, in solving many problems—ranging from cost containment to specialty and the geographic maldistribution of physicians. Some have even suggested that the federal government no longer support biomedical research because it should be the responsibility of the private sector. Another issue of increasing importance, both in health and in other sectors, is the distribution of authority and responsibility among levels of government. President Reagan's New Federalism proposals have brought this issue to the forefront.

In the growing national debate about health policies, more attention must be given to the actual and potential role of academic medical centers, also called academic health centers. These institutions are the loose confederations of medical schools and their affiliated teaching hospitals, which often have dental, nursing, and pharmacy schools as well as graduate academic programs as integral parts of their enterprises. Research, health professions education, and patient care have been their central functions.

Academic medical centers educate our physicians, dentists, pharmacists, and many of our nurses, and they set the pattern for the practices of these professionals. They staff teaching hospitals, and indeed frequently build and operate them. Academic medical centers also are major providers of health care. They have a virtual monopoly on the most sophisticated medical technologies and procedures. In addition to caring for patients referred for highly specialized services, many academic medical centers are the principal providers of medical and dental care for their surrounding populations. Many of those needing the services of the medical centers are poor and lack the means to pay for health care. Academic medical centers have also been the home of the health profession's elite—professional societies, licensing boards, accrediting boards, and other important bodies. In addition, the leaders in academic medical centers have commanded the ear of national and state policymakers as well as influentials in the private sector. In short, the influence of the academic medical center is pervasive in determining the character and cost of health care in the United States.

For the past thirty years, the academic medical centers have responded to federal and state policy initiatives related to biomedical research, health manpower development, health planning, and the financing of health care. These policies are now undergoing dramatic, and, in some cases, drastic change. New ideologies, values, priorities, and constraints are directing attention to academic medical centers. Thus, pressures on these institutions from diverse sources can be expected to increase, particularly in relation to efforts to limit rising costs. Under these changing circumstances, it is appropriate to raise questions about the future role of the academic medical center.

> Occupying as it does a position of great power in the American health care system, how well does the academic medical center fulfill national needs in relation to research, health manpower development, and health care?
>
> As health policies change to reflect national needs and priorities, how is the academic medical center likely to respond?
>
> In the health care system of the future, how will the academic medical center best serve the public interest?

To consider these questions, it is useful to begin with a brief look into the past. The seeds of the academic medical center were sown before World War I with the Flexner Report, but they did not begin to grow until after World War II, when the federal government began to support biomedical research in medical schools and universities. Support for biomedical research has had a profound effect not only on research but also on health professions education and health care. Support for biomedical research was only the first step by the federal government in its support for programs intended to create, nourish, and sustain academic medical centers. In the early 1960s the federal government took another major step and committed itself to the direct support of health professions education. Many states followed suit by expanding existing schools or creating new ones. These policies were sustained and expanded well into the 1970s.

In the mid-1960s the enactment and implementation of Medicare and Medicaid had a profound impact on the health care system as a whole and on academic medical centers in particular, because their teaching hospitals play a major role in caring for the poor. With the infusion of Medicare and Medicaid funds for patient care, federal and private dollars for research, and federal, state, and private support for education, academic medical centers grew rapidly in number, size, and complexity. In part, the growth was in response to public policies. It was also consistent with the internal goals of the institutions. The problems arising today within academic medical centers are partially due to the divergence of the academic goals of the institutions and the demands of society.

The changing policy environment at the federal and state levels has combined with fiscal strain at the national, state, and local levels and the continuing rapid increase in the costs of health care to create unprecedented pressures on and opportunities for academic medical centers. These institutions are also beginning to feel the effects of the anti-inflationary policies of the federal government, the current recession, and the cutbacks in government funding at the federal and state levels. Funds for the support of research have leveled off in constant dollars. There has been a sharp drop in federal aid for health professions education. Capitation grants to the schools are coming to an end. There are few, if any, federal dollars for construction or for student aid—particularly scholarship funds for low-income students. At the same time, health care expenditures have continued to increase rapidly, and thus are consuming a growing share of federal and state budgets. While attempting to contain the growth of these expenditures, policymakers increasingly focus on Medicare and Medicaid at the federal level and on Medicaid at the state level—two of the primary sources of support for graduate medical education, teaching hospitals, and the professional fee incomes of medical school faculties. One of the few remaining sources of flexible funds for medical school departments has been the funds generated from faculty practice.

In addition, a variety of measures to contain the rising costs of health care have been attempted in recent years, ranging from voluntary efforts by the hospitals in the late 1970s to mandatory or voluntary cost controls imposed by state governments. The mandatory controls affecting all third-party payers appear to be the most effective. Although these policies have not been directed primarily at academic medical centers, they have had a major impact on teaching hospitals and medical schools.

Although the relationship of the fiscal crisis, the recession, and health care cost containment to the problems facing academic medical centers may seem to be of overriding importance, New Federalism, as noted by Sheps and Lewis, may prove equally important in the long run. New Federalism was the centerpiece of the Nixon administration's strategy to limit federal involvement in domestic social programs and to decentralize programs to state and local control. The policies were meant to strengthen state and local governments by directly transferring revenues from the federal government and eliminating the strings usually attached to federal grants. The Nixon administration instituted revenue sharing to reduce the federal role: general revenue sharing with states and local governments, and special revenue sharing (block grants) in broad program areas such as social services and health manpower training. The Nixon administration had only limited success convincing the Democratically controlled Congress of the virtues of New Federalism. Nixon had no luck at all in the health field; indeed, the number of categorical grants in health increased in the early 1970s and support for health professions education and programs in academic medical centers increased rapidly during that period.

The most dramatic and radical expression of New Federalism is reflected in the policies advocated by President Reagan. In the area of health, these policies include (1) a dramatic reduction in federal support for health professions education, leaving it up to the states to decide what should be done; (2) the consolidation of twenty-one categorical health programs into four block grants with a substantial cut in the funding of these programs; and (3) major federal changes in Medicaid policy, reducing the federal role and providing the states new flexibility to reduce program expenditures.

The changes in Medicaid policy, which are likely to have a tremendous impact on academic medical centers, were incorporated in the Omnibus Budget Reconciliation Act of 1981. This act reduced the federal share of Medicaid funding; altered Medicaid rules for eligibility, benefits, and payments; provided states greater freedom to determine eligibility and benefits for the medically needy, to make hospital payments less dependent on hospital costs (states were no longer required to reimburse hospitals after the services were provided at the Medicare rate); and authorized the Secretary of Health and Human Services to waive a variety of statutory requirements, including freedom-of-choice requirements.

The picture today is dramatically different from that of just a few years ago. The issues and problems facing the academic medical center are complex and will not be easily, quickly, or comfortably resolved. Some hallowed medical traditions will certainly be questioned and some past practices discarded. Clear, objective analysis is needed to address the issues and problems affecting the academic medical center, and few authors are so well qualified to undertake this task as the authors of *The Sick Citadel.* Cecil Sheps and Irving Lewis have been among the keenest minds analyzing health policy developments during the past twenty years. Both have been key participants in the policy process, and both bring to the task formidable intellectual talents and relevant experience in public policy, health care, and health professions. Sheps and Lewis carefully trace the roots of the current problems facing the academic medical center, and they address the issues from the perspective of the public interest, rather than that of the provider or a special interest. *The Sick Citadel* will certainly stir controversy because it proposes major changes for the academic medical center, including an expansion of the center's goals to include community service. The authors make clear their intentions when they say that "the academic medical center must give high priority in its teaching, research and patient-care programs to the major health problems *of the population of its area* and to practice in the community" (Chapter 7, page 227). They propose that the Flexner model, which has dominated American medical education for seventy years, no longer be the sole approach. They favor the health service delivery model that has been tested in Israel (at Ben Gurion University of the Negev) and is being adopted in medical schools in Holland, Norway, Sweden, Poland, and Great Britain. In these schools there is a strong emphasis on primary care and community needs.

The views expressed by Sheps and Lewis contrast sharply with the views of many leaders in academic medicine and others, such as Victor Fuchs, who suggests "Society would benefit from the evolution of a medical care system where academic centers concentrated on research, teaching and tertiary care, and did only as much primary and secondary care as is necessary for them to carry out their principal missions." (Fuchs, *Health Affairs,* Summer 1982).

Even though others may disagree, the views expressed in *The Sick Citadel* deserve to be heard and heeded. The book brings to the attention of health professionals, academic medical center administrators, policymakers, and the public the full dimensions of the health policy problem, and it proposes courses of action that need to be carefully considered by all concerned.

Preface

    This book was written to analyze and draw attention to an inadequately understood phenomenon of our health care system, namely, the role and power of the academic medical center and its fundamental dependence—substantive as well as fiscal—on public policy. Our purpose is also to emphasize the converse point: the dependence of the public upon the academic medical center for the attainment of the goals of overall public policy in health.

The dramatic advances in the biomedical sciences that have been made in this century are widely recognized. The nature and significance of the resulting organizational changes in medical schools, hospitals, and their associated educational and health service institutions are much less appreciated and discussed. These changes are reflected in the new institutional entity, the "academic medical center," or, in its broadest nomenclature, "academic health center." The controlling forces in such centers are the medical school and the hospital; thus, we concentrate our own interest on the academic medical center. In their breadth of scope and influence these centers are uniquely American.

The academic medical center is at the core of the nation's health care system. It feeds it, fuels it, and overtly runs a substantial part of it. It fully controls the most specialized medical care; at the same time, it is the doctor to much of urban America, rich and poor alike. It produces tomorrow's physician and profoundly influences current and future medical practice. It shapes the future of our health services.

Because it has a special relationship to the health care needs of its community and region as well as the public at large, the academic medical center is clearly differentiated from the rest of the university. Functioning in both academic and nonacademic environments, heavily dependent upon federal, state, and even local tax funds, it must live in two worlds. Thus it is faced with certain unique responsibilities and tasks that universities and their faculties do not readily welcome, accept, or cherish.

The universities and the public tend to see the center as an academic research institution, but it is more than that. Its broad range of functions gives it the power to determine the scope, pattern, availability, and cost of health services. Since health services are undergirded by funding from government at all levels, the central health policy issue affecting these centers is not their ultimate financial viability but rather their capacity and willingness to respond to considerations of the public interest as health priorities and public needs change over time. Of course, the special interest of the centers is to preserve their academic strengths as they see them in their own terms. But the public interest, while not necessarily in conflict with the centers' own goals, extends into the nonacademic world of society's health needs and the justification for public subsidies of the centers.

We believe that there is a misfit between the social demands of the time and our health and political institutions. The public posture of the academic medical centers is that they are aggrieved, threatened, misunderstood, and subjected to new demands without adequate resources to meet them. Additionally, they view many demands for service or cost controls as unreasonable and unnecessary. On the other hand, government does not recognize that the academic medical center has become the core of the health care system; its behavior toward the centers does not always consider that they live in the two disparate worlds of the university and the society. Government deals with the center not as a new institution but as a group of independent schools and service institutions, forcing each back to an approach focused narrowly on survival. The real crisis, for government and for the centers, is one of health policy in terms of purpose, organization, and accountability.

In our judgment, the breakdown in the essential relationship of the centers and government and the search for answers require a full appreciation of the historical development of pertinent public health policy and of the functions, organization, and financing of the centers, as well as the problems of relationship between the centers and public policy. This historical development helps to explain not only the behavior of government but also the goals, structure, and governance processes of academic medical centers. To elucidate the critical role of the academic medical center and its relation to government in nonscientific matters, we have discussed in extensive detail both the historical development and the current status of the crucial issues. Such detail is essential, we believe, if there is to be a real understanding of how the essential medical education and scientific research activities of the university are intertwined with an extensive range of patient care and community service functions. Understanding the past helps explain the present and facilitates the development of effective solutions to the problems of the partnership between the centers and the public.

The history of the centers is, of course, full of significant achievements. However, these very achievements and the methods by which they have been made have created problems and challenges for the future which cannot be tackled effectively by the same organization, attitude, and approach that have become the dogma of the present. Facing the future in a fundamental way is not only difficult but produces anxiety, especially on the part of those who are tyrannized by their past role in producing success, as they see it. We have tried to illuminate the key issues that need to be faced if the quality of the partnership between the academic medical center and government is to improve and permit a full realization of its social and academic purposes. Our analysis led us to clear conclusions about what must be done to improve the academic medical centers in modern terms rather than simply to preserve them in their present form.

We hope this book will be useful to two broad audiences. The first group that comes to mind, of course, is medical faculties, the medical profession generally and their leaders, top university administrative officers and boards of trustees, the nonmedical health profession schools, and officials of state university systems. In addition, we look not only to the general public but to persons with broad concern for the public interest in federal, state, and local governments—legislators, executives and their staffs, trustees and executives of the 1,000 teaching hospitals, health insurance companies, health care organizations, and public interest and consumer advocacy groups.

The field of medicine carries much mystery for the general public. Its achievements and its apparent power over life and death have produced deep appreciation and awe. Nevertheless, the public has serious dissatisfactions. These center on the range and scope of control which we believe that it ought to have. Medicine needs to understand that it has a social purpose that goes far beyond the transactions between the individual physician and the individual patient. We have therefore attempted to demystify the academic medical center for the public at the same time as we explain the purpose of public policy for health in our nation. We believe that it *is* feasible for the public to understand these issues and thus to have much more to say about them. After all, if a democratic society wishes to determine the public interest, it must ask the public—and the public cannot avoid responding. We hope also that our colleagues in the centers will find our discussion useful. Without a fundamental reappraisal, major problems will remain unsolved and the partnership will continue to be uneasy and unsatisfactory to both the centers and the public.

As authors, we sought each other out. Each saw in the other a colleague who could complement and deepen his examination of the history, progress, and problems of health policy and academic policy. Each of us came to our involvement with, and interest in, academic medical centers from a different background of training and experience. One was trained in political science, followed by extensive work in federal government policy and finance. This included increasing responsibility in the Bureau of the Budget in Washington with special reference to health and welfare services, and significant administrative responsibility in the Department of HEW, after which he joined the faculty of a medical school as professor of health policy. The other was trained in medicine and public health with extensive experience in hospital and medical care administration, the organization and administration of public health programs, administrative responsibility in universities including the Vice Chancellorship for Health Sciences at the University of North Carolina at Chapel Hill, and research and teaching in several medical schools in the broad field of social medicine. Drawing on this background, our book is based on the direct experience we have had over the years with well over thirty academic medical centers, supplemented by special field visits we made to a sample of a dozen centers to gain additional insight. In addition, of course, we made an extensive review of appropriate documents, reports, and relevant discussions in the literature.

From the start to the finish ours has been a joint undertaking—we share the authorship, the insights, the errors, and what we hope is the wisdom of our product. As authors, only the order of the alphabet ranks us.

Above all, we hope our book will stimulate discussion and debate. Some will say that we simply do not understand the special needs, not to mention benefits, of medical research and education. They may even say that our recommendations are misleading, if not dangerous. We are aware that our views are controversial but we were encouraged to find, as we discussed our analysis with valued colleagues in responsible positions in centers across the country, that we were by no means alone. To those who will say that we are antiscience we respond that, on the contrary, we advocate more science, not less. We urge that more research in social science be added to current health-related research and that research efforts be aimed, more than currently, at the major health problems of the population.

Of course the way of significant change is not easy. In fact it is difficult. As G. K. Chesterton once remarked of Christianity, it is not something that has been tried and found wanting, but rather something that has been found difficult and then abandoned. Neither public policy nor academe can rest upon the laurels of past achievement. There is a new world waiting to be born in health promotion and health care, and in education and in research related to it. We hope our work will help move this process closer to fruition.

Irving J. Lewis
Cecil G. Sheps

Acknowledgments

We owe much to the many persons whom we interviewed at academic medical centers and government agencies and to all those who not only wisely counseled us but made useful comments on the manuscript. We are very grateful to Janie Jenkins, Bonnie Mietling, Patricia O'Donnell, and Patricia Reggio for their unflagging patience in typing and retyping the manuscript and in keeping our travel schedules in order.

We owe a special thanks to The Commonwealth Fund and the United Hospital Fund of New York for their financial support, which helped us to write this book.

Above all, we acknowledge the forbearance and the encouragement of our wives, Ann Sheps and Rose Lewis, to whom we dedicate this book with the greatest of appreciation.

Introduction: Public Policy, Pluralism, and the Academic Medical Center

THE ESSENCE OF THE POLICY TASK

It is now an accepted tenet of American social policy that all citizens, regardless of means and place of residence, should have equitable access to health care. For many years the federal government and state governments have taken steps in this direction. The task of public policy for health in the years ahead is to decide in what way and how quickly this principle of universal access is to be put into full effect. We cannot expect this to be either an easy or a brief undertaking, for it raises large and basic political questions concerning the responsibilities for decisionmaking and the nature of the mechanisms for carrying out those responsibilities. Among these questions, actively being debated in Washington and state capitals today, are the relative roles of the public and private sectors and the federal and state governments.

The health care crisis is not a crisis of knowledge, facilities, health personnel, or money. Rather, it is a crisis of organization, a crisis of planning, a crisis of relationships. It cannot persuasively be argued that we need more doctors or more hospitals or even significantly more money. We are already devoting a greater proportion of our national resources to health care than any other nation, including those that have achieved much greater access to health care for their citizens than we have. Our research establishment is unparalleled. What we now need to do is to find ways of assuring equitable access that are effective and economical.

The great American debate about health care has moved on from two fundamental issues that long engaged our national concern. The first of these issues was the expansion and application of medical knowledge: the improvement through scientific research and development of our ability to prevent, diagnose, and treat illness and disease. The second was the political acceptance of the goal of universal access to the benefits of medical knowledge and medical care.

Research and clinical medicine supported by large public expenditures have dramatically enlarged our capacity to improve people's health status. Meanwhile, the egalitarian drive in our society has brought about a series of legislative enactments incorporating the principle that all Americans are entitled to accessible and comprehensive medical care.

Some, of course, will continue to debate whether such access to health care is a right or a privilege. We believe the question is now moot. Our political attitude about the responsibility of government for the welfare of its citizens has changed radically during the past fifty years. In the 1930s, the assurance of an adequate income to the aged and the infirm was a revolutionary concept. But that ideal was in time translated into our own social security pension system, which is today as American as apple pie. We are now well on the way to a similar consensus on the assurance of adequate health services. The United States is the last of the Western industrialized societies to have come to this political agreement.

The critical issues that we must now begin to address are of a different—and perhaps even more difficult—nature. We will face even thornier questions of values in adjusting differing relationships and interests in our society so that equitable access to health service becomes a reality. And these adjustments will be all the more troublesome because of growing restrictions on increasing our resources for health care.

General economic constraints, accompanied by high rates of medical price inflation, have today made the control of costs and the limitation of spending almost the overriding policy imperatives at all levels of government. Costs can be most effectively controlled, however, within the context of a national health program that reflects the interdependence of the various parts of the health care system. We do not yet have such a program.

The need for coherent, coordinated policies and for logical structure and order in the health system derives from the requirements of the patients, not the health providers. Comprehensive care of the patient necessitates a systematic relation between his physician and various other physicians, nurses, technicians, hospitals, and other supporting health institutions and services. We take these arrangements for granted and assume that the professionals will see to them.

But health services are not manufactured commodities transported over long distances to meet consumer demand. Rather, they are locally produced by resources already in place. Therefore, it is the interaction of available manpower, hospitals, and payment mechanisms that determines whether people actually have access to proper care at the proper time. If the medical education component of the health system continues to train mainly highly specialized personnel while the insurance component favors inpatient care over ambulatory care, the impact is dual: more hospital services, fewer primary care services.

The fact is that the usual competitive market forces do not work in health, and particularly not if we wish resources to be distributed to meet social as well as economic goals. It is the physicians who make the basic decisions about what kind and level of health service to use. Insurance then insulates the patient from the economic consequences of these decisions.

If resources are relatively finite and are to be directed to meet social as well as individual economic goals, policies governing the number and type of hospitals have to be coordinated with similar policies affecting manpower. Both should then be fitted to the sources and methods of payment. Otherwise, gaps in service remain, costs escalate, and duplication occurs. Above all, equity of access is seriously compromised.

NATIONAL PRIORITIES IN HEALTH POLICY

Our experience with diverse health policies since the 1960s amply demonstrates that equitable access to health care will not be achieved by a series of unconnected measures by government and providers. Public insurance for the elderly, private insurance for the public at large, subsidies and grants for the poor (Medicaid)—all have been helpful in strictly financial assistance per se. When Medicare was enacted, it was not expected to relieve the elderly entirely of the financial burden of health care. Contrary to the popular perception, Medicare today pays only about 45% of the medical bills for the elderly. The new financing progams, unfortunately, have contributed substantially to continued cost escalations, so that the elderly's out-of-pocket expenditures for health care today represent about the same share of personal income—20 percent—as they did in 1965. [1]

Strategies for a massive expansion of biomedical research dominated the federal health policies of the 1950s and the 1960s. While, to be sure, this effort has enormously expanded our ability to diagnose and treat disease, our use and misuse of the resulting technology has had not only a substantial financial impact but also an unhappy social cost. The fragmented health care system of post-World War II America has become even more disorganized, overspecialized, and depersonalized. Both access to and continuity of care have suffered as a result.

We have also greatly expanded the infrastructure of our health care system—hospitals, nursing homes, manpower. Though, of course, this growth was meant to meet "community needs," specific targeted planning was vague at best, especially for nursing homes and health personnel. In the case of hospitals, where the Hill-Burton Act called for general adherence to state and regional plans, the criteria applied have proved to be based on grossly exaggerated estimates of need. Substantial growth in numbers of doctors and numbers of hospital beds occurred when physician specialization increased. At the same time, doctors and hospitals followed the postwar population movement into the suburbs, while major urban medical institutions stayed behind in deteriorating cities and competed feverishly for individual survival. The decrease in the number of primary-care physicians was accelerated. In our rush to introduce new technology, we duplicated expensive facilities, services, and equipment. As a consequence, we now must pay the budgetary and organizational price of a general excess of resources in doctors and hospitals.

In growing recognition of the deficiencies of public programs which were directed separately to individual parts of the system, we tried to stimulate state and local health planning as well as demonstrations of comprehensive health care delivery and regionalization of services. But they have turned out to be too modest in their goals, too small in scale, and too removed from related policies and programs. And, most important, they have been altogether dependent on the voluntary participation and cooperation of the health care professionals and institutions. Inevitably, such attempts at coordination and planning have had little impact upon the larger delivery system as a whole. Successor programs developed in the 1970s continue to suffer from many of the same in adequacies. As Robert S. Lynd said over forty years ago in his book *Knowledge for What?*, "our brilliant technological skills are shackled to the shambling gait of an institutional Caliban." [2]

In summary, as with so many other serious domestic problems, our public policy for health has been one of limited, modest, even tentative interventions or increments. The incrementalist approach, or the "science of muddling through," derives from our American political traditions and carries much appeal. But it is inappropriate to the times and to our present problems in health care. These problems are too massive and too interrelated to be solved by small interventions taken independently. Even if the intervention itself is substantial, the fact that it affects individual and distinct programs or sets of institutions makes it likely to be ineffective as well as costly.

Despite our great advances in education, research, and hospital facilities, and despite the vastly increased health expenditures which have made them possible, millions of Americans live today with inadequate medical care. Our greatest need now is for primary care, the sort of care that is most seriously lacking in urban as well as rural areas. In fact, much of this need reflects the dual effects of past public health and medical successes. Because people now live longer, they are eventually afflicted with degenerative and chronic diseases which require particularly extensive individualized services. There is a vast and growing technological misfit between our public needs in health care and the facilities and services that are provided. Our system has become biased towards elaborate and expensive hospital care and payment for specialist services.

Our national priorities in health policy highlight the need to deal with this problem. We have already begun to restrict funds for development of hospital resources, manpower, and even research, all of which had been lavishly supported by federal and state funds. Forecasters now anticipate an oversupply of doctors by 1990 to accompany our already recognized oversupply of hospital beds. Tomorrow's focus will not be on increased numbers of doctors, but on their appropriate distribution by geography and specialty. Similarly, it is now expected that any national health insurance plan would be accompanied by programs to improve health care delivery, to plan and regionalize services, to expand the scope of preventive medicine, to evaluate technology, and to control costs.

In fact, no part of our health care system can be viewed as an island. Doctors, hospitals, medical schools, and medical laboratories are inextricably intertwined with each other as well as with government policies and subsidies, Medicare and Medicaid, and health insurance. Developing a system of health services that is accessible and affordable by the nation will depend ultimately upon the coordination, coherence, efficiency, and effectiveness of the system as a whole—and all its parts.

PLURALISM IN THE HEALTH CARE SYSTEM

If the priorities seem to be clear, the way to their achievement is not. Our health care "system" today is a loose structure of many diverse special interests and power centers without systematic and ordered relationships. They come together formally and informally in multiple, distinct decision-making mechanisms that intersect both the public and the private sectors and the three levels of government. Here lie the formidable problems of organization and the adjustment of relationships and interaction that must be addressed in the direct pursuit of our health goals and priorities.

Americans place a high value on the diverse and pluralistic character of the health care system. We have viewed health care as largely a private, personal enterprise in which the public role is limited primarily to helping pay for care for those who cannot afford it and subsidizing the production of resources. No consensus has been reached on the responsibility of government for organizing services or improving our decisionmaking mechanisms in order to implement agreed-upon priorities and carry out desired programs.

In any pluralistic system, of course, no single group or person is in control. Power is divided and shared among a wide range of private and governmental bodies. Each has some influence in deciding how the system functions. Some power centers are strong; others are weak. Not all groups are interested in all issues, but each tries to preserve its own power and thus tends to resist change. Major policy decisions are usually reached by processes of bargaining and alliance making in which not all participants are of equal strength.

By these tests, the American health care system is highly pluralistic and is becoming increasingly so. Neither the number of claimants for legitimate participation in the competition for power nor the pattern of interest group relations remains static. They change with advances in science, improvements in technology and patient care, population shifts and economic trends, consumer expectations, patient demands, and a host of other external and internal forces.

The alignment of forces within the health care system was radically transformed after World War II.[3] Until that time, the solo, fee-for-service practicing physician had been the dominant influence in American medicine. He was represented by the American Medical Association, whose views generally prevailed in interactions between the public and private sectors of the health economy. Medical education, philanthropy for research and hospital care, and state and local public health services were the only other visible group interests, but their impact was minor.

Two continuing and mutually reinforcing factors have diminished the power of organized medicine and compelled it to share power with other very large and highly complex institutions. The first has been the extraordinary growth in scientific and technological activity and the manpower education developments that were so generously supported by government biomedical research, education, and other grants. With this support our medical schools have evolved into much larger and more complex institutions to develop and accommodate their ever-growing research interests and the application of rapidly expanding new technology. Simultaneously, hospitals have expanded and became more complex to accommodate the application of these new developments. Thus, they are now multifaceted community resources for the local economy as well as for medical care. Out of this process has emerged the modern academic medical center.

The second factor has been the development of a series of insurance programs, commercial and quasi-public, in addition to government payment programs. As a consequence, the health care system has found itself able not only to meet the rapidly rising costs of specialized, hospital-based medical care but also to offer new services. In particular, the insurance plans permitted hospitals to take advantage of each new technology at little or no immediate cost to the patient.

Today's specialist physician finds himself less in solo practice and more in a maze of referral patterns and organized settings, all tied to the hospital, medical school, and third-party payer. These organizations and their representatives—the Association of American Medical Colleges, the American Hospital Association, the Blue Cross Association, and the Health Insurance Association of America—are our new major interest groups and power centers.

In addition, the specialization of work among health professionals and the development of new types of health workers and services have multiplied the number of participants in the total bargaining process. Nurses, technicians, paramedical personnel, independent practitioners, and other health workers have organized through trade unions and a complex of licensing and accreditation arrangements to protect their own interests and demands.

Another set of powerful forces has emerged in both state and federal government as the traditional limited governmental activities in public health services have been supplanted by hundreds of programs in support of research, education, hospitals, and financing. Now being further enlarged by public as well as public/private health planning agencies at all three levels of government, this heterogeneous government bureaucracy has its own range of priorities and interests. Some agencies are fully allied with other private and public interests; others are quite independent. At the federal level the National Institutes of Health and the Health Care Financing Administration of the Department of Health and Human Services, and the Veterans Administration are the most significant. Since states have many parallel interests with the federal government, they have similar organizations, to which must be added extensive health manpower, education, and mental health structures. In major urban centers the public municipal hospital can be another significant force, as in New York City, Chicago, and Denver.

The general public is poorly organized to participate in this fractionated health system except through the normal political processes of government. Consumer demand for a larger role and influence has been met by a range of responses, from mandated representation in local health planning agencies to the development of consumer-controlled health care systems, such as some prepaid group practices and health maintenance organizations.

The difficulties inherent in the present system can be readily illustrated. Because the costs to society for health care also represent the income to the elements of the system, it is clear that any major government effort at cost containment or control encounters substantial opposition from interest groups. The defeat of President Carter's proposals in 1980 to control and limit hospital costs is a case in point. Although the final proposals would at best have applied to less than 20 percent of the total health care bill, they were ultimately not enacted. No group will voluntarily surrender its share of the $287 billion now going into the system, and we can anticipate acrimonious competition among all groups to maintain their existing shares of increasingly restricted resources within any system of resource allocation.

Independent of the matter of income and costs, the principal interest groups see little to gain and much to lose in the emerging priorities. For example, the medical profession, including academic physicians, opposes measures that would in any way restrict the freedom of physicians to decide in which field to specialize and to choose their practice location. The medical education establishment does not welcome proposals for meaningful and /or large-scale primary care education and training, and accepts curtailment of specialist training only on budgetary grounds, not as policy. Hospitals resist community or regional planning and rally strong local support to oppose the closing of hospitals or limitation of the number of hospital beds. The commercial insurance carriers and the Blue Cross support only such proposed public insurance measures as do not threaten their positions. Finally, the drug and equipment manufacturing enterprises and profit-making hospitals naturally prefer to maintain their own high earnings within the present fragmented but profitable system.

Faced with these clashes of powerful interests, "realists" argue that such goals as redistribution of manpower, expansion of primary care, or control of costs are too ambitious. They say that we will fail if we pursue them and advise us to draw back now. The health care providers and insurance interests are seen as strong enough to defeat any efforts that would threaten their self-interests, from a meaningful national health insurance program to effective local planning and decisionmaking mechanisms.

The realism of such a view is, however, deceptive. It simply avoids the necessity of choice that is imposed upon a society when the national interest clashes with parochial, vested interests. The inescapable reality is that our resources are inadequate to support all special health interests in the form that they have been supported in the past—as uncoordinated elements of a technologically oriented and extremely high-cost system that meets our needs for health care poorly.

On the other hand, there are those who call for a radical departure from present arrangements and a venture into some sort of national health service or system, such as may be found in several industrialized and socialist countries. Although the links among government, patients, and providers might be variously arranged, the essence of such proposals would be to vest unmistakable authority in governmental agencies for all crucial policy, resource, and organizational decisions.

The administrative consequences of such a course would obviously be formidable. Physicians, hospitals, other health care providers, insurance companies — all are opposed to such a government takeover. Most importantly, proposals for a national health service dismiss the manifest preference of Americans for the values of choice and diversity in health services and in the manner in which they are provided.

But public policy can hardly remain stranded. Pluralism exacts a price, and it is dysfunctional if it promotes duplication, waste, and inefficiency in the system, rather than economy and quality through competition. It is unlikely that, in the face of compelling necessity to allocate scarce resources, we will indefinitely allow public budgets to be the hostages of the health care system. Yet popular expectations demand government action. It is worthwhile to ask, therefore, whether there may not be some middle ground, some less sweeping approaches that would encourage coordination and leadership while preserving as much as possible the most valuable features of pluralism.

THE ROLE OF THE ACADEMIC MEDICAL CENTER

Attention must also be paid—and is, in fact, increasingly being paid—to the role and the growing problems of the academic medical center. Sometimes also called a university health sciences center, such an institution is a loose confederation of a medical school, the teaching hospital(s) most directly related to it under its university auspices, and some or all of the health-related professional education, research, and services under the same auspices. Together these centers make up a very special and highly valued set of health care resources and interests. As a complex, it is today our single most important medical institution.

There has been a steady deterioration in the strong alliance between government and the academic medical centers which was forged after World War II. Confrontations over distribution of funds, over policies and programs, over attitudes and even over academic freedom itself, have largely replaced the harmony of this formerly symbiotic relationship. Many public officials, now see the academic medical center as the problem, rather than the solution. On the other side, the medical schools have become wary and fearful that government pressures may lead them down strange and unsuitable roads.

The academic medical center finds itself in a financial predicament. Under more constrained government budgets, the support for education and biomedical research has been moved down on the scale of budgetary priorities. Service programs are often rated higher. But as hospital costs come under closer scrutiny, the reimbursement for teaching hospitals tends to be squeezed toward the average of all hospitals, with inadequate recognition of extra teaching costs. Since their revenues are being cut on both sides, the medical centers see themselves as neither able to continue as they were nor free to support themselves by moving in new directions.

The medical center also finds itself in a programmatic predicament. For some years, public policy has been consistently supporting the expansion of training for primary care physicians while the community has pressed for more primary care services. These demands, of course, run counter to the vigorous allegiance of our medical schools to the training of specialists in tertiary care hospitals and thus to the provision of such specialist services. And yet, when the center does respond however grudgingly, it too often finds itself without necessary support. Both in urban and rural areas, ambulatory or community services are often nonexistent or poorly organized for either manpower training or patient care. In addition, neither government nor private insurance provides sufficient reimbursement for the costs of care of the medically underserved who use these primary care services.

It is no wonder, therefore, that the academic medical center has been described as "a stressed American institution."[4] We ignore at our peril this turn of events in the relationship between government and the center. For although our health system has always tolerated highly diverse interests, it has come to function through the actions of highly organized and institutional forms that move in concentric circles around a common core. That core is the academic medical center, and its health, will determine the health of the whole system.

In expanding the range of its enterprise, the academic medical center has become a big business, but naturally one that requires substantial external support. The 126 centers vary in the scope of their interests, but most have far more extensive undertakings than existed under the more limited research and education focus of the medical schools alone. To manage their networks of schools, hospitals, clinics, laboratories, training facilities, research centers, and other operations, the academic centers have found it essential to introduce some of the techniques and skills of modern corporate management. As a group they employ several hundred thousand people and spend billions of dollars a year. Unlike the business corporation, which must generate its own revenues, the centers must look to outside funding sources for not only their academic functions but also their patient-care services. Both areas require significant subsidy, which can come, in the main, only from government.

At this time, still committed primarily to research and education, the centers remain watchful about the new priorities. As they strive to achieve financial stability in some independent fashion, they may actually frustrate government objectives (for example, by marketing specialist services of questionable relevance which then have the eventual effect of driving up hospital utilization and medical care costs).

If the centers must depend upon government for extensive and continuing support, government similarly needs them—and for much more than research and development. It needs the active cooperation of the centers, strategically located as they are at the heart of the health care system, in order to make any reasonable progress towards achieving the new range of our health priorities.

The public interest underlying government support of medical research extended to health and medicine the scientific successes during World War II achieved with government funding. But today government is looking for much more: institutional leadership in planning and organizing a more coherent health system, provision of services to the medically underserved in inner cities and in rural areas, elimination of unnecessary and duplicative services, and control of technology and costs. Moreover, this search for assistance is led by agencies other than the National Institutes of Health, with which the medical schools have long had a familiar and comfortable relationship.

Consequently, government can no longer accommodate uncritically the aspirations of academic medicine. Instead, asked to support academic medical centers, government must ask how the centers can best serve the public interest in a new set of health priorities. Both government and the medical centers have to contribute to the answer.

Government and the academic medical center are now the dominant, powerful forces in our health care system. The successful operation of the system will be possible only through their active collaboration with each other. Neither the goals of the centers nor the priorities of government can be realized without a continued alliance that recognizes the changes since World War II and anticipates further needed changes. Our purpose in writing this book is to show why this is so, to illuminate the essential character and current status of this partnership, and to recommend the direction of positive and effective change.

NOTES

1. Charles M. Fisher, "Differences by Age Groups in Health Care Spending," *Health Care Financing Review,* Vol. 1, No. 4 (Spring 1980), pp. 78 and 89. Special Committee on Aging, United States Senate, *Health Care Expenditures for the Elderly: How Much Protection does Medicine Provide,* A Staff Paper. Washington, D.C.: U.S. Government Printing Office, April 1982.
2. Robert S. Lynd, *Knowledge for What?* (Princeton: Princeton University Press, 1939.)
3. See Eli Ginzberg, "Health Services, Power Centers, and Decision-Making Mechanisms," *Daedalus,* Vol. 106, No 1 (Winter 1977), p. 204.
4. David E. Rogers and Robert J. Blendon, "The Academic Medical Center: A Stressed American Institution," *New England Journal of Medicine,* Vol. 298, No. 17 (April 27, 1978), pp. 940-950.

Chapter 1

The Evolution of Public Policy
for Health Care

REASONS FOR GOVERNMENT
INVOLVEMENT IN HEALTH

Government is now extensively and irreversibly involved in virtually all medical and health activities in the United States. The public's business is no longer confined to such public health functions as improvement of sanitary conditions or control of epidemics. Instead, current government policies for health encompass the entire health system, private as well as public: the development of resources and the organization, delivery, and the financing of services, as well as the traditional, now greatly broadened, regulatory protection of the public health.

The United States is not unique in its assumption of substantial government responsibility for the health of its citizens. All the Western and industrialized nations of the world have made similar commitments. And in carrying them out, they have inevitably had to confront a long-standing tension within the medical profession between two sometimes conflicting views of the priorities for the health of their citizens. On the one hand, many believe that the first and highest duty of medicine must be therapeutic—to care for and heal those who are already sick.

On the other hand, many see the task of medicine as maintaining and improving the health of all people, not just those who may require immediate treatment. In general, Western societies have been moving steadily toward the latter and more inclusive view, thus extending governmental responsibilities more pervasively to both curative and preventive medical activities.

To be sure, government's far-reaching involvement in medicine is often decried as interference with individual liberty and the free medical marketplace. Yet historically, Western society has never really regarded medical care as just a commodity to be bought and sold on the market, like shoes or meat. It was the medieval church, in fact, which first assumed the duty of caring for the sick and disabled poor, and therefore in a sense established the public, social nature of this obligation. Later, an increasingly affluent bourgeois society was able to supplement the work of the churches with private philanthropy, which again was based upon concepts of social duty and public interest. In our own time, and for a variety of reasons, government has inherited the responsibilities for health care that individuals and social agencies are unable to sustain, ranging from public operation of hospitals and clinics to public payment for private medical care. The consensus is clear: we now believe, as a nation, that no one should be denied medical care because of lack of means. Each industrialized society goes about solving its health problems according to its own political, social, and medical traditions and circumstances, but all countries have taken action to "interfere" with the marketplace. The United States is no exception.

Furthermore, government has other motives for its intervention in the marketplace beyond the inability of some citizens to pay. It undertakes to fill the gaps in service that are left by the independent practicing physician or the private institutions in the society at large. For example, government has historically cared for the mental and chronically ill; for persons afflicted with tuberculosis or "loathsome" diseases; for the elderly who require costly long-term care; and for other population groups for whom the practice of medicine in its traditional form would or could not make adequate provision. Much of this governmental responsibility long preceded the preventive public health measures that government instituted in the latter part of the nineteenth century.

Throughout its history, in fact, government involvement in health care in the United States has been as extensive as the times and resources made possible, given the state of scientific knowledge and technology and the expectations of society. Until the twentieth century, the practice of clinical medicine had had little broad impact upon the health of society. Since that time, government involvement has come largely in response to the medical enterprise's own need for new resources.

Although health care is not a new or unusual area of governmental responsibility, the extent of government involvement today and the rapid growth of government's own health enterprises make our problems different in kind as well as in size from what they were some forty to fifty years ago. For it is indisputable that the federal government—like all the national governments of Western Europe and other industrialized societies—now exercises the dominant influence in the shaping of health policies and health affairs. Three broad forces have brought this about.

First, there has been a relative decline in the fiscal capacity of state and local governments to furnish health services to the poor and to other special groups. The obligation to meet these costs has had to be increasingly assumed by the federal government as other social needs have pressed upon the resources of lower-level governments.

Second, the economic costs of progress in medical science have been high. Extending the benefits of this progress has required an explosive increase in the expenditure of society's resources for health care. This trend has been particularly marked in the transformation of the hospital from a place where the sick poor could die into a twentieth-century technologically oriented institution for the treatment and cure of all classes of people. The increasing financial burden imposed by modern hospital and medical care was abundantly clear even in 1932, when the Committee on the Costs of Medical Care issued its landmark report. We had then hoped to find the resources through commercial and voluntary insurance. This expectation was not fulfilled, and major public programs of financial assistance have since been enacted by Congress.

Finally, the division of responsibilities between the public and private sectors and the high degree of specialization that has accompanied the growth of medical science and technology have created a very complex and fragmented system of health care. Some organizing force is needed to assure the coordination of doctors, hospitals, and other health care providers as well as health care payers. Government, therefore, not only supported the creation of required resources but moved actively into areas of health care planning and organization.

The magnitude of government participation in health-related activities in the United States can be traced most clearly through an examination of national health expenditures. The United States spent an estimated $287 billion for health care in 1981. Public sources, federal, state, and local, accounted for $123 billion, or 42.7 percent of the total.[1] The United States now spends 9.8 percent of its gross national product of goods and services on health, almost a threefold increase over

1929, and more than twice as much as in 1950.² Furthermore, public spending has been increasing twice as fast as private spending. As a consequence, over 10 percent of our total government budget today is for health programs, a doubling in the past ten to fifteen years.³

This high and increasing level of public expenditure has not resulted from a deliberate and systematic policy. On the contrary, as government has moved gradually and incrementally to assume new tasks, it has done so on a highly pragmatic basis, in response to perceived needs and in accordance with the federalism of our Constitution. Health is a major concern of all levels of government: federal, state, and local. In fact, federal programs account for two-thirds of public spending. But while spending for health has risen to 12 percent of the annual federal budget, state and local governments have retained major health functions and their spending has increased to about 9 percent of their budgets.⁴

Our pragmatic policies, however, have not assigned discrete health functions to any of our three levels of government. Consequently, all of them participate in all of the four broad functional health areas: research, education and manpower, the delivery of services, and the protection of community health. Under countless laws—there are several hundred distinct federal health programs alone—government agencies undertake many different activities. They produce and consume health services; they pay for services; they subsidize the construction of hospitals, research facilities, and educational institutions; they regulate and subsidize the supply of manpower and hospitals; they prescribe standards of quality and performance; they undertake research in their own laboratories and support the entire national research effort; and they act as innovators in organizing new health services.

Because health activities are so widely dispersed throughout the three levels of government, it is possible to describe only in broad terms the division of functions within the federal-state partnership. The federal government has become the dominant partner in paying for health care and subsidizing and undertaking biomedical research. Except for the federal veterans' and military health care programs, admittedly very extensive, the state and local governments have the prime responsibility for educating and training health personnel, producing and delivering health services through public facilities and manpower, conducting public health programs, and financing the construction of health facilities. Federal support for these state functions is largely, but not wholly, in the form of financial subsidies, research, and technical assistance. Health planning and service innovations are a shared responsibility, but leadership rests with the federal government.

Nevertheless, the whole structure is characterized by fragmentation, duplication, and overlap because our approach to health policy has been fundamentally categorical rather than comprehensive—categorical as to disease, population groups, type of service, or means of financing. Each new program is typically legislated, organized, and funded separately from existing programs.

This categorical imperative has had significant organizational and programmatic implications for our ability to achieve our national health objectives. It has meant that there is little coordination *within* each level of government as well as *across* levels of government. Because the private sector in health is similarly fragmented in its activities, consensus on public/private sector relationships exists only on the broadest possible, thus vaguest, basis. It is here that we find what we have earlier termed the health crisis in organization.

NINETEENTH-CENTURY DEVELOPMENTS

Public policy for health in the nineteenth century was framed by the basic structure of the Constitution, which created a federal government of enumerated powers, reserving all other powers to the states. Since the Constitution did not specifically authorize any health functions for the new federal government, the states retained their responsibility to maintain and protect the health of the public, and to care for the indigent and other groups not attended to by the practicing physician or charitable groups.[5]

Our first national health legislation was based upon the power of Congress to regulate foreign and interstate commerce. In 1798 Congress created the Marine Hospital Service to provide medical and hospital care to merchant seamen. For many years these services were actually financed by the seamen's own contributions, but after the 1880s the hospital system was financed by direct federal appropriations.

Congress later preempted for the Marine Hospital Service the functions of quarantine and immigration inspection, and vested in it a broad authority to investigate the causes of all communicable diseases and to prevent their spread. In statutes beginning with the 1878 port quarantine act, Congress settled the long federal-state quarrels over the authority to prevent and control epidemics of yellow fever and cholera as well as recurring outbreaks of plague and smallpox. In 1901 Congress also established the Hygienic Laboratory for bacteriological research and public health studies and authorized the surgeon general to call annual conferences of state and territorial health officers. In 1912 the Marine Hospital Service was renamed the Public Health Service, and in time it added to its patient care responsibilities the operation of hospitals for leprosy and narcotics addiction.

Until the middle of the nineteenth century the states did not particularly concern themselves with emerging health matters. Local boards of health and health departments were then organized in order to deal with recurring issues of bad housing, street and public sanitation, quarantine, and the regulation of public nuisances such as slaughter-houses. The 1850 Shattuck report on health conditions in Massachusetts marked the beginning of the public health movement, but it was not until 1869 that Massachusetts established the first state public health department. By the latter part of the nineteenth century the successes of bacteriological research had moved public health concerns beyond the areas of sanitary reform to the scientific control of communicable disease. By 1915 public health agencies had been established in all states, and a new profession had been born.

During these years states, cities, and counties continued to carry on their responsibilities for direct patient care. To the general public hospital, caring mainly for the poor, were added a number of hospitals for special populations or diseases, such as mental illness, tuberculosis, chronic disease, and long-term care. After 1840 the states especially entered the field of mental health, at least in a custodial way, as a result of the humanitarian movement to aid the mentally ill.

These trends and movements in government health affairs proceeded quite independently of the development of personal health care resources and services under private capital or philanthropy. Until bacteriological research and the discovery of anesthesia had made surgery both safe, and painless, hospitals remained largely institutions for the poor. When they became an effective source of medical care, however, the private practice of medicine gradually began to be dependent upon them. In time, a hospital appointment became an essential element of individual medical practice. Hospitals evolved rapidly into the centers of technological innovations associated with surgery and radiology. In 1909 there were 4000 hospitals in the United States, compared with 178 in 1873.

By World War I our health service facilities and the basic organizational structure linking the physician to the hospital had been largely determined. This structure has remained substantially unaltered in spite of the many refinements and adaptations resulting from changes in medical education and training of physicians, the development of scientific knowledge and technology, and the new methods of insurance to pay for care, especially hospital care.

HEALTH POLICY BETWEEN
THE WARS

After World War I the distinction between medical care and public health grew more intense professionally, but it began to disappear in public policy. The war had required the creation of major military health services and had brought about a continuing government responsibility to furnish good medical care to veterans, initially for service-connected disabilities and later for economic disability regardless of service connections. This responsibility led in time to a new and extensive system of government medical care under the aegis of the Veterans Administration. These activities inevitably brought in their wake a broader governmental concern for medical questions.

This enlargement of government horizons in health also took place at state and local levels. With the growth of medical specialization and of hospitals, concern for the quality of care had encouraged the states during the latter part of the nineteenth century to adopt regulatory measures in licensing and accreditation of doctors, nurses, hospitals and other providers of care. The government's own expanding public health services for the poor and for patients with specific illnesses began to overlap the extensive outpatient dispensary services being developed during the 1920s by the voluntary general hospital.

At the same time, government was being urged and propelled to assume more extensive responsibilities in selected fields. Under the Sheppard-Towner Act of 1921, which was officially disapproved by the House of Delegates of the American Medical Asociation in 1922, the Children's Bureau provided federal grants to assist states in developing and administering plans to deal with problems of maternal and child health and welfare. The program was automatically discontinued in 1929 when its authorization expired. In 1928 Senator Neely of West Virginia introduced the first bill for a federal program of cancer research, and two years later Congress changed the name of the Hygienic Laboratory to the National Institute of Health, endowing it with broad research authority.

Even before World War I, the American Association for Labor Legislation had spearheaded a movement for compulsory national health insurance financed by employee, employer, and public contributions. In 1927 the growing recognition of the financial and organizational problems of medical care led a group of foundations to create the Committee on the Costs of Medical Care. In 1932, the Committee's report recommended far-reaching changes in medical practice organization and financing, calling for systems of medical care groups in health centers related to hospitals and financed on a group payment basis through the use of insurance or taxation, or both methods.[6]

It was the enactment of the Social Security Act of 1935, however, and its subsequent validation by the Supreme Court, that marked the clear turning point in national health policy. From then on the federal government's concern for the nation's health was no longer inhibited by a constitutional doctrine limiting its range of action to powers specified in the Constitution. Rather, it could now act under the broader considerations of the Constitution's "general welfare" clause, adopting such health programs as were responsive to felt needs and acceptable to broadly held political values.

Understandably, perhaps, the initial thrust of the new federal policy was to attack discrete problems by making categorical grants-in-aid to state and local governments and nonprofit institutions. The policy was specifically applied in the Social Security Act of 1935, whose broad purpose was to provide protection against several forms of economic insecurity, especially that associated with old age and death. The Act initiated old age pensions financed by employee-employer taxes administered under trust fund arrangements. It also created what was expected to be a temporary public assistance or "welfare" program of grants to states from general revenue, and started two major health programs. Title V of the Act authorized grants to states for maternal and child health activities, and Title VI authorized annual appropriations for grants to states to assist them and their political subdivisions in establishing and maintaining adequate public health services.

The federal government had financed medical care programs as relief measures during the depression after 1933. At that time, compulsory health insurance programs had been considered by the Committee on Economic Security set up by President Roosevelt. Although the committee did not recommend such programs, the question of government's financial responsibility for health care for all its citizens had entered the arena of public debate at the federal level. Our first National Health Survey was undertaken in 1935/36 by the Public Health Service. Subsequently, the Social Security Board initiated ongoing programs of medical economic research. The gathering of population and health statistics through such activities was to bring to public attention wide areas of need, opening the way to discussions about appropriate public policy to fill in the visible gaps in money and services. The first of such debates were held in the National Health Conference of 1938 called by the federal government.

During World War II the needed expansion of the medical services of the defense establishment led to a wholly new understanding by government of the professional and academic leadership in medicine. This appreciation brought the best of the civilian side of medicine to the service of the military and the veteran, leading in time to a total revamping of the Veterans Administration medical care system which made it a significant component of our education, research, and patient care health systems. More significantly for postwar national health policy, World War II brought to the federal consciousness the potential power and prestige of medical research.

TWO POLICIES: THE "CATEGORICAL IMPERATIVE" AND INVESTMENT

After World War II our public policy for health changed fundamentally. The improvement of our national health status became a high social priority, the fulfillment of which led to a sustained leadership at the federal level. At a quickening pace, the federal government became involved in the full spectrum of health activities. Government has now become irrevocably committed to massive expenditures for health care, research, and education, which represent an ever-increasing proportion of both the nation's resources—gross national product—and the federal budget. Federal health outlays in 1965 were $5.6 billion; by 1970, $17.6 billion; and for 1980 they were estimated at about $70.4 billion.[7] Although this policy has evolved on a pragmatic, incremental basis, it has been guided by some overall strategies and an attempt to consider health needs broadly. In November 1945 President Truman delivered the first presidential message devoted entirely to health. It stressed four points: (1) an adequate hospital system, (2) new initiatives and approaches in biomedical research, (3) training of medical manpower, and (4) a national medical care program. (He did not at that time include proposals for a clean environment and other expansions of Public Health Service activities, which a new breed of health planners in the Public Health Service had also proposed to him.)

In 1948 Truman called another national conference of experts, special interests, and representatives of the public to review the status of the nation's health and health services. This National Health Assembly was attended by 800 people, far more than participated in the conference of 1938. Truman's subsequent National Health Program was probably the first full expression of a comprehensive health strategy for the nation. In it he built upon the earlier planning and the information about the supply of hospitals, health manpower, and other health resources that had emerged from the 1948 National Health Assembly to support his proposals for larger medical research and hospital programs, and for assistance to medical schools and medical students. Although the National Health Assembly had not taken a position on government-sponsored health insurance, the National Health Program proposed in 1949 specifically recommended compulsory national health insurance.

In many ways, the government and the nation had readied themselves for this new federal effort. In 1937 Congress established the National Cancer Institute as a focus for national research. In 1939 President Roosevelt moved the Public Health Service from the Treasury Department to the newly created Federal Security Agency, for closer coordination with the activities of the Social Security Board. The 1944 revision of the Public Health Service Act had provided the necessary legislative authority to support an extramural research effort. Scientific activity during the war had opened the way to dramatic progress in the physical sciences and to miracles in the biomedical life sciences. Demobilized servicemen, returning to the universitites to complete their interrupted educations, were looking for opportunitites in research and medicine. And private health insurance was providing new funds for hospitals. Though in 1940 only 9 percent of the population had been covered by voluntary health insurance to pay for hospital care, insurance plans developed so rapidly during the war as a fringe benefit under collective bargaining arrangements that by 1948, 40 percent of the people were so covered.

The country was ready for those measures that would prove to be politically feasible. The major political stumbling block proved to be the issue of compulsory health insurance, which was bitterly and successfully opposed by forces led by organized medicine. The Wagner-Murray-Dingell Bill of 1949 did not reach the floor for debate. (It had first been introduced in 1943.) Neither did any other Truman insurance proposals, and by the early 1950s a clear consensus had developed that voluntary health insurance provided by Blue Cross, Blue Shield, and the commercial carriers was worth a trial. Organized pressure for a compulsory government-financed insurance plan ceased until the early 1960s.

Meanwhile, if "politics is the art of the possible," what Congress found possible—and the executive found acceptable—was the continuation of the "categorical" approach. Over the years a variety of categorical programs developed and expanded to meet specific health needs and purposes. The categorical approach minimized the need for political confrontation and maximized the opportunity for pluralistic bargaining, an opportunity limited only by the availability of federal funds. In view of the relatively steady growth of the American economy from the end of World War II until after the Vietnam War, this proved to be an insignificant limitation, at least for programs that could win broad political support.

The categories that developed seemed to be of an infinite variety.

Some programs were based on *disease* (cancer, heart disease, tuber-culosis, venereal disease, etc.); some on *age* (maternal and child health, national insurance for the elderly); some on *institutions* (hospital or neighborhood health center grants, nursing home loans, school health services and payments to providers of care to welfare recipients, known as vendor payments); some on *geography* or *political* jurisdictions (state health grants or Appalachia health centers); some on *activity* or *service* (research, construction, manpower training, rehabilitation, hospital care, etc.). In time, several categories were combined, such as programs for heart disease, cancer, and stroke, or services for crippled children.

Although each of the many categorical programs did some good, it is surely questionable whether they represented the most effective approach to rationally defined and genuine health needs. Certainly many of them functioned as a surrogate for tackling the basic issues of how to create a rational and efficient health system that would better serve the public interest.

Since each categorical program had its own legislative authority, we ended up with a sprawling, splintered federal health establishment in both the executive branch and the Congress. Not until 1968 did the Department of Health, Education and Welfare, established in 1953, create the Office of the Assistant Secretary for Health to oversee the independent programs of research, manpower, hospitals, and state health services in the Public Health Service and to provide some overall health policy guidance for the Department. Today, efforts still continue to coordinate these Public Health Service activities with the other programs in the reorganized Department of Health and Human Services related to the elderly, the disabled, and the poor or to the reimbursement of health providers. In Congress, responsibility for health has been similarly divided among the health, finance, ways and means, interior, veterans and appropriations committees.

In this context, postwar health policy was heavily shaped by an extraordinary alliance among academic scientists; laymen with the voluntary health agencies like the American Cancer Society, the National Heart Association, or the National Association for Mental Health; professional leaders in major federal health agencies; and the members of Congress. Under the leadership of Mary Lasker, the so-called Health Syndicate focused from the outset on expanding research, but its spokesmen also led the way toward health policy for hospital facilities and health manpower for specialized purposes. Consistently outflanking the executive branch, which was reluctant to exercise leadership in health during the 1950s, Congress molded and shaped postwar health policy under the guiding hand of Senator Lister Hill, chairman of the Senate Health Subcommittees on both legislation and appropriations, and Congressman John Fogarty, chairman of the House Appropriations Health Subcommittee.

By the mid-1960s, it was clear that the categorical approach had run its course as a basis for implementation of national health policy. A new direction was needed. The word "categorical" developed increasingly negative connotations, and new policies, programs, or services were described as "comprehensive." The retirement of Senator Hill in 1968 and the death of Congressman Fogarty in 1967 came at a time when federal budgetary constraints were beginning to compel Congress and the president to examine all health programs in terms of their contribution to the functioning of the overall health system, as well as their individual merit. An era of unprecedented Congressional leadership was coming to a rapid end.

During these two decades one clear principle had emerged as controlling in Congress: if Congress would only undertake to develop further basic health resources, health services would then become more widely available and more readily accessible through the functioning of the "medical care market." Consequently, public policy for health was not only categorically directed but also was conceived in terms of investments.

With the creation of additional health resources as a working assumption, Congress proceeded first in 1946 to subsidize the construction of hospitals through the Hill-Burton program. Next it undertook to develop the country's biomedical research effort through the National Institutes of Health. This guiding policy of investing in the development of resources as the means to improve the nation's health status was articulated by the Senate Appropriations Subcommittee, chaired by Senator Lister Hill, in a statement in 1960:

> There has come into being a national policy that calls for a sustained and expanded research attack against disease. [The effect is to increase] the acquisition of new knowledge which will lead to a more precise understanding of the nature of the many fatal or disabling diseases which afflict our people, thus hastening the day when these may be prevented, cured, or ameliorated.[8]

After it became evident that additional measures were needed, in 1963 Congress granted funds to build medical school teaching facilities, thus inaugurating a new program of investment, to expand the supply of health manpower. But as the 1960s wore on, Congress found it necessary to address directly the question of patients' capacity to pay for health care. Accordingly, in 1965 it enacted the Medicare and Medicaid programs.

The investment policy continued into the 1970s, but since problems of access to health care and of differential health status continued despite the sharp rise in health care expenditures, the government shifted its attention to the organization, delivery, and financing of care, hoping to promote effective utilization of resources. The Partnership for Health Act of 1965, consolidating a number of public health grants and initiating comprehensive health planning for manpower, facilities, and services, had presaged this new concern. By the mid-1970s governmental priorities emphasized a comprehensive approach to the health system and an attempt to rationalize the distribution of resources.

FACILITIES DEVELOPMENT

From around 1930 through the end of World War II, few hospitals were built in the United States. To eliminate the postwar deficit of hospital beds, the Hill-Burton program (Hospital Survey and Construction Act of 1946, as amended) provided a major financial stimulus for the construction of hospitals. As this deficit was corrected, funds were provided for the modernization of hospitals as well as the construction and modernization of both diagnostic and treatment facilities and rehabilitation facilities.

The Hill-Burton program was a federal-state partnership. The federal government formulated guidelines for state planning and for the award of construction subsidies, but the actual operation of the program was directed by state agencies. Before it ended, the program helped 4000 communities build or modernize about 6500 facilities at a total cost of approximately $14.5 billion, of which $4.1 billion was paid by the federal government, the balance coming from state and private funds.[9]

During the twenty-nine-year history of the program, the number of short-term general care beds in the nation increased from 474,000 to 931,000. The ratio of hospital beds to population rose from 3.4 to 4.4 beds per 1000 people.[10] After 1970, the Hill-Burton program shifted its emphasis from grants to loans and loan guarantees, from subsidies for hospitals to subsidies for outpatient facilities, and from rural projects to urban projects. These shifts occurred in part because a national oversupply of hospital beds had apparently developed, potentially leading to unneeded hospital utilization and to increased costs. In addition, new funding sources became increasingly available in the form of reimbursement for depreciation through insurance and the Medicare/Medicaid programs. Such reimbursement enables hospitals to obtain construction loans in private credit markets, especially through the sale of tax-exempt bonds. By 1974 the traditional Hill-Burton program had come to an end, and it was absorbed in a new National Health Planning and Resources program, under which only limited government support for hospital construction is provided.

BIOMEDICAL RESEARCH

The most dramatic and sustained federal investment to develop health resources was in biomedical research. In 1947 federal expenditures for such research were only $27 million, less than one-third of the total national biomedical research expenditures of $88 million.[11] By 1968, when growth in expenditures slowed down, the federal outlay had reached $1.6 billion, and ten years later, after a new growth in funding had taken place, it was $3.8 billion, now more than 60 percent of the total national research expenditure of $6.2 billion. In 1981, federal expenditures were estimated as $4.9 billion of the national total of $8.5 billion.

The National Institutes of Health (NIH) is responsible for about two-thirds of all federal spending for biomedical research. From its modest beginning in 1887 as the Hygienic Laboratory of the Public Health Service, the NIH has become the primary stimulus to and support of the entire national research effort. It now includes fifteen institutes and major bureaus with interests covering the spectrum of medical science and its technology. In 1980 the NIH spent $3.2 billion for health research and development, about 40 percent of the national effort.

This expansion did not take place without political controversy. In 1945 fundamental issues of public policy divided the scientific community and the government establishment on how to build on the wartime progress that government had financed under the direction of the military Office of Scientific Research and Development headed by Vannevar Bush, president of the Massachusetts Institute of Technology.

To begin with, there was the basic question of the role of government and its potential control over science. Related to this general issue was the further question of whether government should support scientific research on a broadly undifferentiated basis, taking its cue from scientists on what activities to support, or tie its support to public purposes, such as health, atomic energy, or defense.

The advisability of substantial government financial support was generally acclaimed, but the university and other research scientists were fearful that government would try to interfere with their scientific investigations or otherwise abridge their academic freedom. On the other hand, government was equally concerned about the accountability of researchers for the expenditure of government funds for publicly established purposes in accordance with fiscal standards normally applicable to government agencies.

Much of the debate in the late 1940s revolved about the public or private character and the organizational structure of any scientific research agencies that legislation then under consideration might establish. And, of course, existing federal agencies, such as the National Institutes of Health, argued strongly for "mission-related" research. After President Truman vetoed a major science bill on the grounds that it would have created a private agency immune from public control, the president and the Congress resolved their differences and established a public agency, the National Science Foundation, with concerns for science in general.

Meanwhile, the growing popularity of health as an area of political action had led many congressional leaders to form an alliance with health researchers, including senior NIH staff, and citizen lobbyists to press for independent action in respect to biomedical research. Thus, when the Office of Scientific Research and Development was terminated, its continuing contracts with nongovernmental scientists for medical research were transferred to the NIH, where they formed the base for budgetary and programmatic expansion. The framework for this expansion was in the legislation under which the National Cancer Institute had been created in 1938: the focus on a disease or problem-oriented activity, the support of research in nonfederal institutions, the award of fellowships to selected scientists, and the establishment of an advisory council of outside scientists and lay leaders. Administrative practices had already been established by NIH for the system of "peer review" by committees of scientists to assure the scientific merit of proposed research projects.

Over the next few years Congress moved rapidly, enacting legislation to round out the NIH research authorities and increasing appropriations each year. By 1950 Congress had added the National Heart Institute, the National Institute of Mental Health, the National Institute of Dental Research, the National Institute of Arthritis and Metabolic Diseases, and the National Institute of Neurological Diseases and Blindness. Each institute was eventually provided with identical authority to subsidize research, including basic research, and research training, specialty and subspecialty training, and disease control, as well as authority to carry out research in the NIH's own laboratories. The central NIH directorate supplemented each institute with funds for additional research support, such as construction of research laboratories, exchange of library information, and encouragement of the work of young scientists.

Until the mid-1960s the expansion of the nation's biomedical research enterprise was lavishly supported, and its central position in national health policy remained unchallenged. For over twenty years NIH commitments and awards grew steadily. By 1969, when budgetary curtailment began, NIH annual appropriations had reached $1,118 million, compared with $35 million in 1950.

The benefits for medical research were significant. The nation developed a comprehensive research activity spanning all branches of medical science. It added greatly to the supply of trained researchers and to medical knowledge, and opened the way to remarkable technological developments in patient care. Moreover, the steady flow of funds into medical schools and their teaching hospitals substantially altered medical practice by supporting the training of specialists and creating specialized clinical care units.

But the expansion of research also had other, less salutary effects. By 1965 54 percent of all funds spent by medical schools was derived from federal grants and contracts, principally from the research and training activities of the NIH. Because of this dependence upon research grants, medical school faculty shifted their interest dramatically from educational activities to research projects. In the process, the NIH project awards to individual investigators seriously fragmented the faculty and weakened the central managerial capacity of the medical school. Moreover, as teaching hospitals and faculty focused increasingly on specialized, tertiary care services for the acutely ill hospital patient, medical educators showed less interest in primary care, chronic illness, and the other medical care problems that were becoming of increasing concern to government and society.

Changes outside the medical school were also taking place. The costs of medical care had begun to mount, in no small measure as a result of the wider use in hospitals of technology flowing from the research enterprise. Medicare and Medicaid were enacted in 1965 to help the public meet these rising costs. But national health expenditures continued to increase at a rate of about 10 percent a year, totaling $47 billion in 1966, 6.3 percent of the gross national product, compared with $13 billion in 1950, 4.5 percent of the GNP.[12] Over half the annual growth was due to medical price inflation itself. Accordingly, in 1967 President Johnson called the nation's health leaders to a National Conference on Medical Costs to see whether costs could not somehow be lowered without impairing quality. Although the conference led to no immediate action, it was a prelude to the future health policy debates.

The 1960s was also the period when other social demands, including those to improve access to health services, began to move higher on the scale of public policy priorities. Thus, two years before the conference on medical costs, after enactment of the Medicare health insurance program for the elderly, the president had convened the White House Conference on Health. His statement to the Conference and its subsequent report made clear that investment in research alone would not be enough to improve general access to medical care, to fill the gaps in service to the poor and other groups with special problems, and to decrease infant mortality and increase life expectancy. The Conference believed that other measures would be needed if we were to "assure that the fruits of our research efforts reach those who provide health services." Thus, the conference concentrated on how to meet needs for health personnel, health protection, and the organization and delivery of health care.

The budgetary demands of the Vietnam War and the new Great Society programs interrupted the growth of NIH appropriations for several years. In the 1970s, however, with the new initiatives in cancer and heart disease and creation of the new Institute on Aging, appropriations again rose rapidly.

Of course, investment in biomedical research continues to be an important federal policy. But biomedical research is no longer the central focus of national health policy, and the level of support for research in general and categorical institutes in particular will tend, in the future, to depend upon a sharper competition for federal funds.

HEALTH MANPOWER

The third federal investment in health resources—the supply of physicians and other health personnel—was slow in coming. In 1950 the country had 220,000 doctors of medicine and osteopathy. In 1953, the President's Commission on the Health Needs of the Nation reported that the 233,000 physicians anticipated in 1960 might actually represent a shortage of nearly 59,000 physicians.[13] But the AMA disagreed with the Commission and successfully opposed programs to support under-graduate medical education directly. Federal aid to general higher education at that time was very limited, and the states were proceeding on their own to open new public medical schools. At the same time, research and post-M.D. specialty training were substantially funded through the NIH.

By 1963, however, the fact of a physician shortage had been endorsed by the American Medical Association and the Association of American Medical Colleges, and was elaborately set forth in reports by a number of new study groups and commissions. While precise agreement on the magnitude of the shortage was difficult to secure because of widely differing assumptions and forecasting methodologies, the figure of 50,000 emerged eventually as the recognized estimate of the probable shortage.

Whatever the actual number might be, this shortage reflected several significant trends. The most important was that medical practice was changing rapidly because of the expansion of the nation's hospital system and the growth of research and technology. Physicians were preferring to become specialists with a dominant interest in hospital care. Fewer and fewer doctors were available for general patient care in the community. The construction of more hospitals generated a further need for hospital-based physicians, particularly as house officers to staff the hospitals. And patients, in turn, were increasingly turning to the hospitals for their ordinary outpatient care. Finally, the demand for medical services was growing as health insurance became more available.

Meanwhile, although the increasing affluence of the country was heightening the desire of young Americans for the educational opportunities in medicine, medical school enrollments were not noticeably expanding. The number of medical school graduates in 1960 was 7,081, only 236 more than the number of graduates in 1956. More and more, the country's need for physicians was met by graduates of foreign medical schools, who were soon entering the United States at a rate of approximately 7,000 a year. The influx of alien physicians raised serious foreign policy questions, especially to the extent that this "brain drain" came from developing countries that were being aided under our economic assistance programs. It pointed up, however, the inadequacy of our own medical education programs.

In 1963, Congress enacted the Health Professions Educational Assistance Act. From the outset, the Congressional intent was clear and direct: to expand, rapidly and significantly, the education and training capacity of health profession schools in order to keep pace with the growth in medical research and hospital care. Expanding the supply of doctors remained the central and most dramatic justification of the new legislation. However, the programs that evolved under later legislation covered other health professions as well—nursing, dentistry, veterinary medicine, podiatry, optometry, pharmacy, public health, and the broad range of allied health professions. Responsibility for the program was first placed in NIH, but in a few years a new Bureau of Health Manpower was created in the Public Health Service, reflecting the emergence of manpower policy as a separate focus of government concern.

In 1965 the House Commerce Committee specifically declared that there was a need for a 50 percent increase in the number of new physicians by 1975—from 7,500 to 11,500 graduates—and for a corresponding increase in places in first-year medical school classes.[14] At first, the funds authorized by Congress were limited to matching grants for the construction of teaching facilities and to loans to students. In subsequent amendments, however, Congress added operating funds tied to commitments to expand school enrollment. For several years, over half of the nation's medical schools received substantial federal "financial distress grants." These grants helped to cushion the effect upon medical education of the declining rate of increase in NIH research funds. Through "special project" institutional grants, Congress also supported the expansion and modification of curricula; it further supplemented student loans with limited scholarships aimed to ensure an adequate supply of applicants.

By 1970 Congress had accepted the argument of the medical schools that they were a national resource. Accordingly, it put into effect a new program of capitation grants designed to underwrite the twin objectives of (1) expanded enrollments and (2) dependable financial support for medical education without reference to the "back door" of research funding.

From 1963 to 1978 the federal health manpower program spent over $6 billion, over 50 percent of which went to aid medical schools and medical school students.[15] By any quantitative measures this activity achieved its Congressional purpose. The goal of increasing the number of new physicians by 50 percent was actually reached in 1974. The increase in number of schools and in medical school graduates continued to grow after 1974 but has now begun to level off.

The expansion of physician supply occurred so rapidly that as early as 1974 Congress and the administration began to worry about a possible future surplus. That the aggregate supply of physicians is now adequate has been attested to in the 1978 report of the Department of Health, Education, and Welfare to the president and the Congress, and is now a generally accepted fact.[16] The 1980 supply of 444,000 physicians projected in the report exceeded not only the original 1971 Congressional goal of 436,000 but even the Department's current estimate of requirements for 1980. The Department also forecast that there would be about 600,000 physicians in 1990—a ratio of 242 physicians per 100,000 persons, compared with a 1960 ratio of 144/100,000.[17]

Against this background, the 1976 Congressional health manpower legislation severely restricted the opportunity for foreign medical graduates to enter the United States and stay indefinitely as part of the physician supply. The assumption, however, that American graduates will naturally fill the residency positions in mental and other public hospitals formerly occupied by foreign physicians, raises its own set of questions.

But if the number of our physicians is now adequate, their distribution is not. In terms of both location and specialty or type of practice, there still exist wide gaps in available medical services. Government had asumed that expansion of supply would tend to direct physicians where they were most needed. Our policy on geographic and specialty distribution was summed up in 1974 by Assistant Secretary for Health Charles Edwards, who testified that:

> If large enough numbers of health professionals are produced...competitive pressure would force them to practice in non-metropolitan areas and in the medical specialties that offer lower income potentials, longer working hours, and/or relatively lower levels of prestige.[18]

This, however, did not happen. In fact, despite a 33.3 percent increase in the supply of physicians between 1963 and 1976, geographic and specialty maldistribution has worsened. It is this problem of maldistribution, not supply of manpower, that is the central concern of current federal policy affecting medical education and training.

Physician shortages in rural areas became more visible as physician concentration in metropolitan areas increased. About 75 percent of the population of the United States now lives in metropolitan areas. By contrast, in 1976, almost 87 percent of active physicians were in such areas, compared with 79 percent in 1963, and the ratio of physicians to population in rural states like Mississippi was only one-third of that in an urban state like New York. In general, physician supply in urban areas has increased twice as fast as in rural areas. There is now a greater dispersion to smaller cities and towns but this masks the continuing shortages in urban ghettoes and rural areas.[19]

The most significant trends in M.D. specialty distribution relate to primary care, that is, the health maintenance and general prevention services usually provided in doctors' offices and other non-hospital settings. Only 39 percent of active physicians were in primary care in 1976, compared with 42 percent in 1963, despite the large increase in supply. This decline would have been even steeper but for the continued movement of young physicians into the specialties of internal medicine and pediatrics, which also render some primary care services. But the proportion of physicians in general practice and family practice has fallen from 27 percent to less than 16 percent. Simultaneously, there are more than adequate numbers in some medical and surgical specialties.[20]

Even while Congress relied mainly upon an increase in aggregate supply to meet the nation's needs for physicians, it had attempted at the beginning of the 1970s to employ other manpower measures aimed at evident maldistribution problems. These included rural preceptorships for students, forgiveness of student loans in return for commitments to practice in manpower shortage and underserved areas, area health education center programs sponsored by medical schools, training of new types of health practitioners, and organization of the National Health Service Corps and award of NHSC scholarships. Independent evaluations have concluded that these measures did not work well or were only marginally successful, a confirmation of the judgment of the Senate or Labor Committee and Public Welfare in 1974:

> The resolution of specialty distribution has been left to our educational institutions and specialty societies, but these bodies have not been given the tools to achieve these results. The problem of achieving a more reasonable geographic distribution of health professionals has been attempted by providing loan forgiveness and repayment features to encourage graduates to practice in a shortage area. The result has been unsuccessful.[21]

In fact, within the free enterprise market, there are few good tools available. The full effect of the National Health Service Corps and scholarship program, committing the medical student to primary care service in underserved areas, is not yet clear. It appears likely that the Congress will have to consider measures more directly restricting career choices if health services are to be made available more equitably. Such measures would have enormous implications for medical schools and specialty societies. Congress showed its awareness of this possibility in the 1976 debates on manpower legislation, which led ultimately to the establishment by the secretary of health, education and welfare of the Graduate Medical Education National Advisory Committee. GMENAC was charged with making recommendations to the secretary on the present and future supply of and requirements for physicians, their specialty and geographic distribution, and methods to finance graduate medical education. One interim report was submitted in April 1979. The final GMENAC report, discussed in subsequent pages, was transmitted in September 1980.

THE HEALTH INSURANCE DEBATE: MEDICARE/MEDICAID

Toward the end of the 1950s, political attention returned to questions of government insurance to help patients pay for the cost of health care. The idea of compulsory health insurance had first been debated before World War I. During and after World War II, the American Medical Association had successfully opposed each proposal of President Truman's, which had been embodied in a series of different versions of the Wagner-Murray-Dingell bills. Unable to secure widespread public support for comprehensive national health insurance, President Truman abandoned the fight by 1950; the issue of government support for social health insurance on a broad-scale basis was laid aside for some years.

Nevertheless, the years of debate had brought about consensus on the wisdom of group payment for health care bills. Blue Cross had been founded during the depression by a group of Texas teachers with the support of the local hospitals; The subsequent growth of private and commercial health plans, was stimulated by their use as a fringe benefit for collective bargaining under the wage freezes during World War II and the Korean War. Group insurance grew so rapidly that by 1958 about 65 percent of the population had some form of coverage, primarily for hospital bills.[22]

Doctors and hospitals fought as fiercely for their financial and programmatic independence from the private insurance plans as they had struggled against the "socialized medicine" of government-financed proposals. They successfully resisted proposals for external cost control and peer review measures, limiting private insurance to a philosophy that its role was simply to protect the insured to the degree specified in the insurance plans. Thus, the commercial insurance companies followed the approach of paying the insured person an indemnity or a fee schedule for specific services, and Blue Cross reimbursed hospitals their "reasonable" costs. The Blue Shield Plans started as service benefit plans in which the physician accepted a fixed fee only for low-income patients, other patients paying the doctor's charges in full, with Blue Shield making only partial payment. In time, physicians moved *experimentally* to the concept of the usual, customary, and reasonable (UCR) charge, paid in full by Blue Shield regardless of the patient's income. By its adoption under Medicare in 1965, the UCR method has become the most common form of fee-for-service payment.[23] Even with the UCR method, however, many insurance plans do not prevent the physician from charging the patient amounts not paid by the carrier.

The early government efforts to move from the investment strategy to the new financing strategy reflected this philosophy, i.e. new insurance programs would be designed merely to pay the medical and hospital bills of the patient, not to alter the system of medical practice in any way. There was no attempt to "disturb" the system by affecting its organization or the quality of medical care. Government ceased its efforts to secure universal and comprehensive coverage, proposing instead to act upon the well-known categorical basis and to recognize that payment for health services was a proper assistance to those special groups that received the continuing attention of the federal government. For the poor on public assistance, Congress in 1957 authorized the use of federal cash assistance grants to pay physicians, hospitals, nursing homes, and other providers of health care. These payments to so-called "vendors" of medical care provided the base for large state welfare medical programs, especially in New York, California, and other states with major public assistance populations.

A second group of special federal interest was the aged. In 1958, only 43 percent of the population over 65 had some form of health insurance, compared with 65 percent of the population overall. Naturally, commercial carriers were not anxious to initiate coverage of the elderly because of their extensive use of health services. But the political lobby for the aged won increasing recognition through special conferences on the problems of the aging and through new legislative proposals. In 1960, to ward off the growing demand for larger insurance benefits for the elderly, Congress enacted the Kerr-Mills program, authorizing grants to states to pay the medical and hospital bills of the "medically indigent"elderly, i.e., those who had adequate resources for normal living but were unable to meet the costs of hospital and medical care.[24]

The health insurance debates in the 1960 presidential campaigns were based on different assumptions from those in 1948 and 1949. First, the concept of medical indigency had become legislatively recognized, even though it was being applied only to one group. Second, the states had become much more active in paying for medical bills for the poor and thus had large budgetary interests at stake. Third, organized labor had begun to accept that it could not secure sufficiently broad coverage of the working man's health needs through collective bargaining that led to private insurance plans. Consequently, labor had moved to support development of a broad national health program, embracing not only financial but also organizational considerations.[25]

Finally, certain deleterious effects of the known advances in medical education and medical care were beginning to be felt. The increased specialization and fractionation of care were making it more difficult to obtain, even for those who could pay for it. In addition, specialization had been accompanied by increases in the costs of care. As medical care prices rose about twice as fast as the general cost of living, they fell heavily upon the elderly.

Demand for and expectation of medical care increased, but so did frustration about what came to be called the "delivery of care." While the interaction of these trends had been evident to the Committee on the Costs of Medical Care in 1932, it was only in the early 1960s that a political force had finally developed that could act upon it, namely the aged. The burden of increasing costs fell most heavily on them, and this was recognized in the 1960 campaign for the presidency.

In many ways, the aged became the cutting edge of public policy. The story has been amply documented.[26] As an ever larger portion of the population, they have increasing importance as a political force; moreover, they have more illness, require more complex care, and use more health services. Implicit in the Kerr-Mills program was the notion that elderly people on fixed and low incomes should not have to worry about where they could get health care. Ultimately it was the provision of health insurance for the aged that allowed government to become involved in supporting health services without reference to the income of beneficiaries.

More than any other program, Medicare established the popular concept that health care is a right. This came about in large part because Medicare is part of the social security system, financed through payroll taxes on employee and employer alike. The principle of "earned right" underlies the original social security pension system, its later extension to the income needs of the disabled, its further extension to the medical needs of the elderly, and most recently (1972) to the medical aspects of disability and end-stage kidney disease. With the enactment of Medicare, the social security system became the preferred method of financing government-sponsored health insurance.

And so the "ideological Rubicon" was crossed by the Medicare/Medicaid legislation of 1965.[27] The Social Security Amendments of 1965 made no attempts to alter the existing patterns of service delivery. In fact, the law disavowed any attempt to interfere with the existing practice of medicine. But proposals for basic reorganization of the health care delivery system and changes in methods of reimbursement could not long be delayed after the passage of Medicare and the corresponding program for the poor, Medicaid. In Medicare, the government applied on a uniform national scale the prevailing practices and techniques of the private insurance industry, treating hospitals and doctors separately. In Medicaid, it left to the states freedom to apply different systems of vendor payments within state plans developed under federal minimum requirements of service; these plans permitted, in fact encouraged, very comprehensive care.

Before long, the cost estimates of the original Medicare/Medicaid proposals had proven to be far too low. If the health system remained in its status quo, government would eventually have to face the difficulties that could be avoided only by a systems approach: excessive price and cost escalation, inadequate services for some covered populations, geographical inequities, and financial fraud and abuse. By 1969 and 1970 the term "health care crisis" had secured wide currency, and even a conservative administration began to propose measures to control the allocation of resources and introduce system changes to link financing and organization of care, such as health maintenance organizations.

Health care prices continued to rise twice as fast as the cost of living. The consensus developed that the health cost problem could be solved only by improving the system itself. A larger understanding of the health system had evolved, in which (a) research and development, (b) investment in capital plant and manpower, (c) payment for services, and (d) rational organization of care were all seen as interrelated. The investment strategy had not achieved the public goal of reasonable access to care. Neither would a strategy limited to financing payment of bills.

PLANNING, COMPETITION, AND COSTS

Over the past fifteen years while consensus apparently developed on the need for a unified health policy, actual policy development has been uneven. With some exceptions for disabled persons, no further progress has been made on a national health insurance plan. Since 1975, the debates on national health insurance have lost momentum. But proposals continue to emerge across a spectrum that includes government-financed and/or operated plans, varieties of mixed government and private schemes, and periodically revised "catastrophic" insurance plans.[28]

Meanwhile, since the early 1960s, the federal government has inaugurated numerous new or experimental demonstration programs designed to affect the organization and delivery of medical care, especially primary care. These activities of neighborhood health centers, family or community health centers, children and youth centers, community mental health centers, group practices and health maintenance organizations, and the National Health Service Corps of health professionals to work in underserved rural and urban settings, were launched outside the legislative and organizational framework of the Medicare and Medicaid programs. Varying state, local, private, or academic medical center sponsors were utilized. Efforts were also begun to develop local health planning institutions and to regionalize services or education in heart disease, cancer, and stroke.

Many factors have contributed to the unevenness of health policy development. One, of course, is that public policy for health is part of overall social policy, which has itself been uneven for some years now, a marked change from the progressive movements of the post—World

War II years. There is an evident national disillusionment about the capacity of government to solve complex social problems and, in fact, even to govern. A rather steady search for definition of the public interest has been replaced, with alarming speed, by a social attitude of concentration on individual gratification of persons or special interests. As our national confidence is shaken, we talk less about justice and more about liberty and "practicalities." We review the history of the Great Society in a context not of ideals but of limits and realism which we presumably previously ignored. And we seem to feel that the major issue of health policy is the control of the national health bill. Health cost containment is seen as a pre-condition to the adoption of further health insurance plans; this issue has come to dominate all public debate, and has severely limited substantive debate on health policy.

Concern about rising health costs certainly has substantial justification. Total national expenditures were $287 billion in 1981, 9.8 percent of our gross national product. The Health Care Financing Administration has forecast that expenditures will reach $438 billion in 1985 (10.5 percent of GNP) and $758 billion in 1990 (11.5 percent of GNP). The projections assume no major changes in our current institutional and inherently inflationary arrangements for payment to providers. But they likewise assume no relief of the consequent financial burden to consumers who have inadequate or no health insurance coverage.[29]

Until recently, health sector inflation had generally far outstripped the rates of general inflation. In 1978, 68 percent of health service expenditures were due to rising health prices, only 25 percent to increased and more intensive services, and 7 percent to population growth. In 1973, when the Economic Stabilization Program was in effect, the comparable figures had been 43 percent, 50 percent, and 7 percent.[30]

Rising health prices not only affect all consumers, providers, insurers, and employers but also have a serious impact on government budgets. Because government pays for over 40 percent of all health expenditures in our mixed public/private system, where expenditures are to meet "uncontrollable" entitlements, the test of each new health program modification is often whether it will help to control or contain costs. For example, the need to match program goals with costs was recognized in the National Health Planning and Resources Development Act of 1974 (P.L. 93-641, Section 1502), wherein Congress provided for a system of some 200 health planning agencies to plan services and to begin a process of regulation and regionalization of hospital services and high-cost technology.

In a gloomy national atmosphere of increasing skepticism about the capability of government and a deepening concern that public budgets have become the hostage of health care costs, the policymaker has

UNIVERSITY OF WINNIPEG
LIBRARY
515 Portage Avenue
Winnipeg, Manitoba R3B 2E9
DISCARDED

desperately turned both to planning mechanisms and to the forces of competition. Blithely ignoring the fact of unequal personal incomes in the society and the historic quest for equity of access, the economic analysis of the free market economist attributes our difficulties to government funding of insurance, either by direct programs such as Medicare, or to tax subsidies for employer-financed private insurance policies. And so we now find a strong government interest in policy prescriptions based upon free market considerations. These usually involve increasing the patient's cost sharing and leaving the fee-for-service system of payment largely intact, since it is assumed that price rationing will control the "uncontrollable" level of health care expenditures.

PLURALISM AND EQUITY

How we move, politically and administratively, to achieve these three priorities of cost control, planning, and competition will have great implications for the academic medical center. It is unlikely that substantial progress toward government health objectives can occur without major support by the academic medical center. A major question is whether the centers will approach these priorities so as to meet the public interest or to protect their own survival. When the Council of Teaching Hospitals (COTH), the hospital branch of the Association of American Medical Colleges, met in May 1980, those institutions were urged to assess the imminence of competition in their communities and prepare to enter the marketplace now; "like it or not," open price competition among hospitals was said to be inevitable."

In our opinion, this is not sound advice. The appeal of competition is illusory, for it fails to deal with the issue of equitable access to care, which must be the eventual measure of the costs and benefits of public policy. But therein lies the politician's dilemma: equitable access to health care requires some form of regulation or infringement upon the individual rights of health providers. Cost or price control is obviously one form of such regulation.

If we are to continue the historical trend toward equality which is the characteristic of Western society since the nineteenth century, there must inevitably be restrictions upon persons and institutions with greater wealth and power, a classification that surely includes the academic medical center. We have not yet imposed extensive restrictions on the freedom of the medical profession, medical schools, and hospitals. While restriction of this "cottage industry" would be administratively difficult, the reason for our noninterference is deeper.

UNIVERSITY OF WINNIPEG
LIBRARY
515 Portage Avenue

Medicine deals with issues of life and death. The popular faith in the power of high-technology medicine to cure and to sustain life remains a powerful opposition to any efforts to restrain the application of technology.[32] How else does one explain the enactment in 1972 of a national program of kidney dialysis despite its obvious high cost? Highly specialized and technologically oriented medicine has achieved the highest prestige, a result to which medical research and medical education have undeniably contributed.

In a sense the American political process deals with the medical profession as it deals with the military.[33] Each profession is treated with great deference by Congress; few questions are raised about the experts' judgement of national needs or their profession's ability to meet these needs. These professions both ask the apparently critical questions and command the production of the imperfect and imprecise data. Both tend to develop excessive technology, which becomes rapidly obsolete.

The steady increase in federal health and other social expenditures has not been confined to particular political administrations. In fact, it reflects a number of structural elements in the political process which reflect certain weaknesses in Congress, the strength of outside special interests, and thus the essential pluralistic environment in which health policy is made.

First, the multiplicity of Congressional power centers has increased the power of narrowly focused special interests. Health and medicine are dealt with by four major House committees (Ways and Means, Interstate and Foreign Commerce, Government Operations, and Appropriations), and three major Senate committees (Finance, Human Resources, and Appropriations). National health insurance and cost containment legislation is the province of two committees in each chamber.

Second, the upper levels of the federal civil service are manned by scientific and professional specialists, whose careers tend to be tied to the Congressional committees and to the outside interest involved.

Third, between World Wars I and II, federal social programs were developed by federal grants to states and municipalities, leading in time to direct and strong alliances between particular federal and state bureaucracies, which became, in turn, supported by the organized lobbies of state and local governments like the Council of State Governments or the National Association of Counties.

Fourth, the post—World War II programs went the nongovernmental route. They followed the pattern that had been created by the military Office of Scientific Research and Development, i.e., government contracted with or granted funds to individuals and to private institutions, rather than to governments. In health and medicine, for example, this pattern produced the alliance that developed between the

National Institutes of Health and the nation's medical schools. After the enactment of Medicare, there developed analogous alliances between the Social Security Administration and the Blue Cross/Blue Shield or other fiscal "intermediaries."

In summary, we find that medicine has flourished within a pluralistic and deferential political environment that has promoted the influence of the scientist and the specialist. In turn, this influence has brought great intellectual and financial support to doctrines of research, experimentation, and demonstration of the value of medical technology. Over time, this influence has become concentrated in the academic medical center. Thus, we now turn to an examination of its development, its tasks, and its role in society.

NOTES

1. Robert M. Gibson and Daniel R. Waldo, "National Health Expenditures, 1981," *Health Care Financing Review*, Vol. 4, No. 1 (September 1982), Table 1.
2. *Ibid.*
3. N. Piore, P. Lieberman, and J. Linnane, "Financing Local Health Services," in *Health Services: The Local Perspective*, ed. A. Levin. Academy of Political Science, 1977, Table I, p. 20.
4. *Ibid.*
5. For an extended analysis and historical review, see Oden W. Anderson, *The Uneasy Equilibrium: Private and Public Financing of Health Services in the U.S., 1875-1965*. New Haven, Conn.: College and University Press, 1968.
6. Committee on the Cost of Medical Care, *Medical Care for the American People, The Final Report.* New York: Arno Press and The New York Times, 1972.
7. Includes health outlays in federal budget functions other than "Health," e.g., Veterans Administration and military hospitals. Source: staff of Health Care Financing Administration.
8. Stephen P. Strickland, *Politics, Science and Dread Disease: A Short History of United States Medical Research Policy.* Cambridge, Mass.: Harvard University Press, 1972.
9. Cambridge Research Institute, *Trends Affecting the U.S. Health Care System*, prepared for U.S. Department of Health, Education and Welfare. DHEW Publication # HRA 76-14503, October 1975, p. 92.
10. Institute of Medicine, *A Policy Statement: Controlling the Supply of Hospital Beds. Washington, D.C.: National Academy of Sciences, October 1976, p.2.*
11. Data on National Institutes of Health are primarily from the series *Basic Data Relating to the National Institutes of Health* (updated annually), Washington, D.C.: Government Printing Office.
12. Robert M. Gibson, "National Health Expenditures, 1978," *Health Care Financing Review* (Summer 1979), p. 3.
13. President's Commission on the Health Needs of the Nation, *Building America's Health*, Vol. II. Washington, D.C.: Government Printing Office, 1953.
14. U.S. House of Representatives, Committee on Interstate and Foreign Commerce, *Current Health Manpower Issues*, Committee 96-IFC-34. Washington, D.C.: Government Printing Office, October 1979, p. 5.
15. Bureau of Health Manpower, Health Resources Administration, Public Health Service, U.S. Department of Health, Education and Welfare, *Manpower: A Change in*

Course, Annual Report Fiscal 1978. Washington, D.C.: DHEW Publication No. (HRA) 79-41, p. 2. U.S. General Accounting Office, *Are Enough Physicians of the Right Type Trained in the United States?,* A Report to Congress. Washington, D.C.: General Accounting Office, HRD 77-92, May 16, 1978, p. 5.

16. U.S. Department of Health, Education and Welfare, *A Report to the President and Congress on the State of Health Professions Personnel in the United States.* Washington, D.C.: DHEW Publication No. (HRA) 78-93, August 1978, p. I-3.
17. Bureau of Health Manpower, *Manpower: A Change in Course,* p. 3.
18. Testimony of Assistant Secretary of Health C. C. Edwards, 1974, cited in *Current Health Manpower Issues,* p. 14.
19. Annual AMA report on distribution of physicians, cited in GMENAC staff paper, *Supply and Distribution of Physicians and Physician Extenders.* Washington, D.C.: DHEW Publication No. (HRA) 78-11, 1978, pp. 34ff.
20. *Ibid.,* Table 2, p. 6.
21. C. E. Lewis, R. Fein, and D. Mechanic, *A Right to Health: The Problem of Access to Primary Care.* New York: John Wiley and Sons, 1976. *Current Health Manpower Issues,* p. 13.
22. Anderson, *op. cit.,* p. 173.
23. J. Showstack, B. Blumberg, J. Schwartz, and S. Schroeder, "Fee-for-Service Physician Payment: Analysis of Current Methods and Their Development," *Inquiry,* Vol. 16, No. 3 (Fall 1979), pp. 230-246.
24. Anderson, *op. cit.,* p. 153.
25. I. G. Falk, "Proposals for National Health Insurance in the U.S.A.: Origins and Evolution and Some Perceptions for the Future," *Health and Society/Milbank Memorial Fund Quarterly,* Vol. 55 (1977), p. 172.
26. For example, see Anderson, *op cit.,* pp. 172-193; Richard Harris, *A Sacred Trust* (Baltimore: Penguin Books, 1969.); and Theodore Marmor, *The Politics of Medicare* (Chicago: Aldine Publishing Co., 1973).
27. Wilbur Cohen, "Policy Planning for National Health Insurance," *Health in America: 1776-1976.* Washington, D.C.: U.S. Department of Health, Education and Welfare, DHEW Publication No. (HRA) 76-616, 1976.
28. *Ibid.,* p. 175; Falk, *op. cit.,* p. 161.
29. M. Freeland, G. Calot, and C. Schindler, "Projections of National Health Expenditures, 1980, 1985, and 1990," *Health Care Financing Review* (Winter 1980), pp. 1-27.
30. R. M. Gibson, "National Health Expenditures, 1978," *Health Care Financing Review* (Summer 1979), pp. 1-36.
31. Association of American Medical Colleges, *Weekly Report* No. 80-21, May 28, 1980.
32. E. Ginzberg, *The Limits of Health Reform: The Search for Realism.* New York: Basic Books, 1977, p. 170.
33. For an extensive review of these issues, see Don K. Price, "Planning and Administrative Perspectives on Adequate Minimum Personal Health Services," *Milbank Memorial Fund Quarterly/Health and Society,* Vol. 56, No. 1 (Winter 1978), pp. 22-52.

Chapter 2

The Academic Medical Center

The dramatic and rapidly accelerating advances in the biomedical sciences that have taken place in this century are widely recognized. As a consequence of these advances, medical schools and hospitals have undergone radical transformations, most notably in the past thirty years. A new institutional entity, "the academic medical center," has been born. The nature and significance of these organizational changes are much less appreciated and understood than are the scientific advances.

DEFINITION AND CONCEPTS

The academic medical center is at the core of our health care system. It feeds it, fuels it, and overtly runs a substantial part of it. Each center is big and complex, employing thousands of people; many centers spend much more than $100 million per year. As the most important and indispensable element in our health care system, the academic medical center has a special relationship to the needs of the public at large and to its community and region, which differentiates it clearly from the rest of the university. It is thus confronted, ineluc-

43

tably, with unique tasks that universities and their faculties do not readily welcome, accept, or cherish.

The public posture of academic medical centers, and their ability to handle the challenges that they must meet today, are rooted in their historical development. Their history explains their present goals, their structure, and the manner in which they make decisions about which programs to initiate and how to conduct them.

In the nineteenth century, medical schools in the United States conducted their educational programs with little or no reference to hospital work. Similarly, hospitals saw little need to be involved in medical education in any way. Today, in striking contrast, there is a great and growing recognition among hospitals, especially the larger ones, that responsible functional involvement with a medical school's education program is crucial to their ability to provide high-quality and complex care. At the same time such involvement enhances the hospitals' prestige with the medical profession and the public.

This new development began to take hold early in this century, when our medical schools began to site and center their entire clinical education program in what came to be known as the teaching hospital. At about the same time, awareness was growing that the quality of medical education depended crucially on the incorporation of medical schools as organic elements of the nation's universitites. By the middle of this century, it had become most difficult for a new free-standing medical school to become accredited unless it was part of a university. The confluence of these developments has led to the concept and organization of the present-day academic medical center—and to its present problems.

The academic medical center must be distinguished from two other kinds of institutions—the medical center and the academic health center. The term "medical center" has been used for about fifty years without a singular and consistent meaning. Some hospitals and some physicians in group practice or even solo practice use the expression to suggest a site where modern medical care, perhaps even comprehensive, is available. In fact, the medical center may be no more than a conventional hospital or a local professional building. The "academic medical center," in contrast, involves a university site with a coordinated organization for formal undergraduate and graduate medical education, biomedical research, and patient care.

The recently coined term "academic health center" has come to denote an even broader set of health activities under a university aegis. After World War II, the programs of education for an increasing number of health professions were moved into universitites so that they might become stronger academically. During this period also, many additional programs were established for existing health professions and for newly developing professions and technologies, almost all in universities and colleges. As these programs grew in number, size, and complexity, many universities grouped them into a single unit for administrative purposes. Such a grouping is often called an "academic health center." The term is commonly used when the university operates a medical school, a teaching hospital, and at least one other health profession school. The academic health center may include dentistry, pharmacy, nursing, public health and the "allied health professions" such as physical therapy, occupational therapy, medical technology, and physician's assistants. The Association of Academic Health Centers, a national organization, include eighty-seven such centers, and there are twenty-eight additional institutions with fairly comparable activities.[1]

Thus the academic health center is larger and more complex than the academic medical center, which includes only the medical school, its affiliated teaching hospital(s), and the university. When this aggregation is part of an academic health center, it continues to consider itself as an academic medical center, and often uses this term. The units in the academic health center are not equals. The size and prestige of the academic medical center make it the most powerful. The presence of other health profession schools and research programs in a joint administrative framework presents opportunities and problems for the medical school and for the other components of the academic health center. However, since our focus is on the interdependence of public policy and academic medical centers per se, we shall concentrate our analysis and discussion on this entity. Without denigrating the special roles of the other health professions in relation to policy, the university, health care and health status, we believe the central issues of public policy, as well as the university's role with respect to health, revolve around the medical school and its association with hospitals.

THE MEDICAL SCHOOL IN PRE-FLEXNER TIMES

A brief review of the historical development of medical education in the United States will reveal the crucial elements underlying yesterday's achievements and today's problems and dilemmas, from which emerge the present and future challenges facing the academic medical center.

In the nineteenth century, there was no single generally accepted and enforced pattern of medical education. At the beginning of the century, training was generally received through apprenticeship to a practicing physician. The apprentice helped the physician in many ways, including sometimes helping look after his horse. Medical education was incidental to participation in the provision of medical care. By the latter half of the century, training was often conducted by independent proprietary institutions set up by a few physicians; these schools offered a purely didactic program that lasted one or two years, and included no clinical exposure or involvement for the student. In some instances, the student was not even required to attend in person as long as he completed the prescribed examinations successfully. In this type of program, medical education was totally unrelated to medical care in the formal educational process.

These medical schools were very unstable. There were several hundred of them in operation at various times in the last half of the nineteenth century, many closing after a few years. They relied for their financial support primarily, if not always fully, upon tuition fees paid by their students. The prevailing situation was typified by what Abraham Flexner found in Chicago and Maryland in his 1909 survey. Of the fourteen medical schools in Chicago, only four had any connection with a university, only one of which he could describe as "integral." The sole financial resources available to eleven of those schools were student fees. Some were clearly commercial enterprises, owned by an individual or operated by a stock company. After surveying the seven medical schools in operation in the state of Maryland, Flexner concluded, "At this date the John Hopkins University is the only academic institution in the state capable of conducting a modern medical school."[2]

Large-scale and fundamental changes have taken place since the early years of the twentieth century, gradually picking up sweeping momentum which led to the domination of a radically different pattern after World War II. These decisive changes in medical education are characterized by a profound reliance on the development of a scientific and academic base, the distinctive professionalization of the faculty within the university setting, and the development of bedside teaching. Because bedside teaching required a close relationship to the delivery of medical care, medical schools developed a controlling influence on the quality, organization, and cost of medical services generally. As a consequence of these developments, the cost of medical education has risen.

It is important to recognize that these decisive changes took place largely through influences external to the medical schools themselves. At the turn of the century, two major external forces—organized medicine and the state licensing boards—produced a growing appreciation that something needed to be done about the low standard of medical education in the nation and the overproduction of graduates by the 160 or so medical schools in operation at that time. The American Medical Association, concerned about the low prestige and earning power of physicians and the prevailing mediocrity of the medical schools, recognized the value of making major improvements in the medical schools. It formed a permanent Council on Medical Education in 1904 headed by Dr. A. D. Bevan. The next year this Council invited the state licensing boards to a national conference to review the status of medical education and to set minimum standards. By 1907 the Council was classifying the schools into categories designated A, B, and C, on the basis of their ratings, and the rate of school closings increased.

But more drastic action was in the offing. Dr. Bevan sought out Henry S. Pritchett, president of the Carnegie Endowment for the Advancement of Teaching, to request that this foundation, whose major interest was education, sponsor a study of medical education in the United States and Canada. Dr. Abraham Flexner, an educator who was not a physician, undertook this study. His professional background was considered to be an asset for this task. Flexner visited the 150 schools in person, and his report discussed, in detail, the history and current status of medical education for each school. This landmark document, popularly known as "The Flexner Report," was published in 1910.[3] It was written with brutal candor.

The report directly attacked the commercialization of medical education. It found that there was an enormous overproduction of uneducated and ill-trained medical practitioners from the commercial schools. However, it also found that the universities had failed to appreciate the great advances in medical education being made elsewhere, especially in respect to the scientific basis of medicine and the necessity to assure high-grade teaching at the hospital bedside. In brief, Flexner's report was as much an attack on the universities for failure to enhance educational standards as it was upon the commercial operators for using low standards to begin with.[4]

Flexner's recommendations were based in large part on the types of schools in operation at that time in Europe, especially Germany, and on the medical school at Johns Hopkins University. His major recommendation was that medical education be grounded much more in the basic biomedical sciences which were than beginning to develop rapidly. He viewed the integration of medical schools with universities as necessary for this purpose. In his judgment this was not to be a nominal affiliation. He saw the university as responsible for applying appropriate academic standards in the medical school and for adequate funding.

Flexner also made the radical recommendation that the curriculum be related much more intimately and continuously in the last two years of the four-year program to hospital experience, including laboratory work. This led to the concept of the teaching hospital, controlled by the medical school, as a major foundation for its education program. Medical education was to become intimately, continuously, and inextricably related to the delivery of medical care in teaching hospitals. Soon after the publication of this report came the proposal, which Flexner supported, that scientific medicine could best flourish in medical schools if their faculties were paid annual salaries so that they could devote themselves fulltime to carrying out their academic responsibilities.

IMPLEMENTATION OF THE FLEXNER REPORT

The relevance and logic of Flexner's recommendations did not produce immediate general agreement.. It was not until after World War II, some four decades later, that this pattern was fully implemented throughout the nation. In 1900 there were 160 medical schools in the United States, enrolling 25,171 students; 5214 students graduated that year. Thereafter, the schools began to decrease in number, with closings accelerated after the Flexner report. The number of schools fell to 76 in the 1930s and remained at about that level until the early 1950s when it began to rise. In 1951, 79 schools enrolled 26,186 students and graduated 6135.[5] Implementation of Flexner's major recommendations was greatly facilitated by the Rockefeller Foundation, which distributed over $78 million for this purpose among the medical schools of 24 universities in the period 1911 to 1928. This helped to finance the establishment of a new medical school at the University of Rochester and facilitated major reformations at schools in such universities as Cornell, Iowa, Vanderbilt, Chicago, and Washington at St. Louis. Since philanthropic funds were not as readily available to them, state governments began to appropriate more tax funds to upgrade the training of physicians being educated in state universities.

Implementation of the radical reforms recommended by Flexner, starting slowly for the following two decades and then accelerating rapidly, especially after World War II, made America a leader in medical education and research in the developed world. The salient feature of this development in the United States was the tremendous and unprecedented expansion of federal support for biomedical research after World War II. Federal expenditure for such research rose from $74 million in 1950 to $1.66 billion in 1970, with 49.5 percent going directly to medical schools. In 1963 federal research funds accounted for 41 percent of the total revenue of the nation's medical schools, but this proportion fell to 30 percent by 1970 as new public sources of funds developed.[6] Although this large infusion of funds was also a hidden subsidy for medical education, production of physicians did not increase for many years. Higher research productivity benefited the science and practice of medicine generally, and also improved the quality of medical students, as Flexner had predicted.

So large were these funds, so prestigious was the conduct of biomedical research, that such activities have come to play a predominant role in our medical schools. This pattern is not unique to medicine. Throughout American universities, particularly in all branches of science, the new importance of research has led to a pronounced shift of emphasis away from teaching. The massive growth in biomedical research, centered as it was among the faculty of our nation's medical schools, has significantly affected the nature of medical education and the goals and priorities of the medical school faculty. The effects have been of mixed value. Less emphasis was given to teaching the undergraduate medical student, and more to the research process and to recruiting and developing faculty whose major interests and skills were in biomedical research. It was argued that the conduct of research improves the quality of the teaching. While this view took hold among the growing basic science faculty, it also quickly led to a new type of professionalization of clinical faculty. The new set of values moved them into basic as well as clinical research. The clinical faculty were now perceived as quite different from the skilled practitioners who devoted all their time to patient care within and outside the hospital. The latter type of practitioner gradually became alienated and "second rate" in the value structure of the medical school.

During the same time that our medical schools were taking on a much larger share of the nation's rapidly increasing biomedical research effort, the role of the teaching hospital in education became fully established, creating a much greater identity of interest and interdependence between the medical school and the hospital. Medical schools intensified the actual participation of medical students in the direct patient care activities of the hospital; instead of learning primarily from bedside rounds conducted by faculty, students now were assigned clinical clerkships in which they participated, under supervision, in the actual care of patients. At the same time, the medical schools confined the clinical learning experiences of the student to hospital patients alone, with the predominant emphasis on the patients sick enough to be confined to bed.

Along with these developments, the hospital began to assume responsibility for graduate medical education in the specialties. Before 1920 only a few major university centers had attractive graduate programs for interns and residents. As late as 1911, the Massachusetts General Hospital had no "house officers." But as the technology of medicine expanded, the hospital increasingly became the focus for graduate education, creating more residency programs especially targeted to advance clinical training in the developing specialties within surgery and medicine. The term "teaching hospital" came into vogue to distinguish hospitals with residency programs from other hospitals even though many of them were not initially affiliated with a medical school.

It soon became clear that applicants for residency positions much preferred hospitals affiliated with medical schools. Affiliation with a medical school became more attractive to hospitals. Since 1960, the role of the medical school in residency programs has been greatly enlarged and strengthened. Whereas in 1964—1965, less than 50 percent of the programs offering graduate training positions were associated with a medical school, this proportion rose to 91 percent ten years later.[7]

At the same time, because much of the supervision of the medical student clerkships and the teaching were conducted mainly by the residents on the specialty services, the medical schools became interested in additional affiliations to support their growing enrollment. From 1946 to 1978 the number of first-year enrollees in medical schools nearly tripled, rising from 6060 to 16,134 with most of the growth occurring after the early 1960s. Residency programs also grew rapidly, reflecting not only the standardization of graduate medical education but also the value of residents in the delivery of care. By 1974 over 57,000 residency positions were being offered under more than 4600 residency programs, more than double the number of positions offered twenty-five years previously.[8] As the activities of their various clinical departments became more specialized and research oriented, the faculty had to seek additional clinical opportunities. Furthermore, given the rapid advances being made through the medical faculties' expanding biomedical research efforts, large general hospitals saw close working relationships with medical school faculty as a valuable means of incorporating the most recent scientific developments in the clinical services available to their patients.

Gradually, as it became clear to hospitals that the most modern specialist care became available most readily by affiliation with a medical school, the public also came to assume that the quality of care was superior in teaching institutions. General agreement developed that medical schools should extend themselves for this purpose to as many hospitals, and even to out-of hospital programs, as possible. This backing of public opinion expedited the change in medical education so that today, in contrast to the past, it is intimately and continuously involved in, and dependent upon, patient care.

Affiliation arrangements between medical schools and hospitals were not always easy to develop. Complex questions of institutional control and autonomy of separate governing boards were difficult to settle. Nor were the medical staff of hospitals united in their views of the value of education as a hospital mission or the methods of achieving this in terms of their autonomy vis-a-vis the medical faculty.

The intimate connection between medical education and patient care is the primary raison d'etre of the academic medical center. There are now 126 centers--at least one in each of forty-four states. New York, Illinois, Texas, California, Ohio, and Pennsylvania have five or more. As expected, the centers have a strong metropolitan flavor--New York City alone has seven, and Chicago and Philadelphia each have five. Several other cities each have two or three such centers.[9]

INCREASING GROWTH AND INFLUENCE

In view of the large-scale development of research in medical schools and the expansion of diagnostic and treatment services representing the application of new knowledge requiring new technology and more highly specialized personnel, it is not surprising that the expenditures of medical schools should have risen very sharply. In 1947—1948, the nation's seventy-nine medical schools spent a total of $70.6 million. Of this amount, $17.1 million, (24 percent) was for sponsored research. By 1965—1966 the expanded activities of the eighty-seven schools then in operation resulted in total expenditures of $882 million—more than an elevenfold increase—on the average. This included $418 million for sponsored research, which now represented 47 percent of the total.[10] By 1978—1979, 112 of the 114 accredited schools reported a total expenditure of $4.8 billion, of which $1.08 billion was for sponsored research.[11]

The diversity of activities now conducted under the aegis of medical schools is very much greater than a few decades ago. These activities include a much greater range of responsibilities than those that are undertaken by any other unit of the American university. While it is generally believed that the interaction among these diverse efforts improves medical education, this relationship is less obvious in some cases than in others. Problems of balance among various activities also arise even though each may very well be worthwhile in itself.

Since the modern medical school is engaged in a very wide range of activities, many of them undertaken jointly, the rise in expenditures is only partly related to rising costs of medical education and to increased student enrollment. The medical school is a classic example of the "joint production" process and resulting "joint costs." It deploys its human and material resources to produce distinctive outputs: education, research, patient care, and community service. Education itself comprises different outputs; for example, M.D.s and Ph.D.s are major educational outputs, but medical school faculty also spend substantial time teaching residents, nurses, and other health professionals. Since much of this process of production is joint—e.g., patient care and teaching of both residents and undergraduate students are carried by the faculty simultaneously—the costs of production are joint and not susceptible of precise determination.

Revenues flow into medical schools from a number of public and private sources, and are expended on a range of general operating programs or sponsored and restricted activities for *all* the products of the schools. Accordingly, the task of calculating the cost of undergraduate medical education, especially for purposes of public policy, is most complex and difficult. The best recognized effort of this type was carried out in 1974 by the Institute of Medicine, National Academy of Sciences. This study reported a range of costs per undergraduate medical student from $6,900 to $18,650, by applying various formulas to faculty-reported costs. Using different formulas the Association of American Medical Colleges reported a much higher range—$16,000 to $26,000.

Whatever the exact costs of education may be, the medical schools of the nation currently represent a major, large-scale financial effort. Exclusive of the budgets of the affiliated or owned teaching hospitals, medical school expenditures totaled $4.82 billion in 1978-1979. The smallest budget was $6.9 million, the largest $114 million, and the median almost $39 million. Student fees supply a very small fraction of the revenues of the schools, only 5.4 percent in 1977-1978—2.9 percent in public schools and 8.2 percent in private schools.[12]

As medical school activities have enlarged, there has been a dramatic increase in the financial support by federal agencies such as the National Institutes of Health, the National Science Foundation, the Atomic Energy Foundation, the Department of Defense, and the Bureau of Health Professions (and its predecessors) of the Department of Health and Human Services, formerly Health, Education and Welfare. The proportion of medical school revenues obtained from the federal government rose steadily from the 1950s to a high of 55 percent in 1965-1966. By 1970-1971 it had dropped to 45 percent, after which it continued to fall to 32 percent of the total in 1976-1977. The absolute level of support did not decrease, however. On the contrary, funds from federal sources totaled $1.269 billion in 1976-1977, compared with $481 million in 1965-1966.[13]

Meanwhile, state governments sharply increased their direct support of medical education in the state universities. In the past decade many state governments also provided per capita support to finance the admission of state residents to private medical schools. State and local government funds have also increased both absolutely and as a proportion of the overall revenues of public and private medical schools, rising from $143 million (16 percent of the total) in 1965-1966 to $1.058 billion (27 percent) in 1976-1977.[14] For the 1978-1979 school year, forty-three states (not including local governments) and Puerto Rico made available $1.080 billion to medical schools located in their jurisdiction.[15]

States have traditionally supported medical education directly, while the federal approach has been one of subsidy. In both cases, government recognized that medical schools are crucial to the further development of health services for the nation and to the implementation of the principle of equitable access to care. Government at all levels has been primarily interested in supporting an increase in the number, the quality, and distribution of physicians, not only geographically but also by type of specialty. By 1960 eleven states were still without a medical school. By 1970, all but six states had at least one medical school. Of the sixteen new schools established in that decade, fourteen were public, and only two were private. The number of accredited medical schools grew from 79 in 1950 to 124 in 1977-1978. Developments such as these, and related activities and trends in the delivery of health services, have been set forth in greater detail in Chapter 1. They are briefly outlined here to indicate the degree to which medical schools, because of the public functions they have undertaken and regardless of their auspices, are deeply and inevitably involved in, and affected by, public policy in the field of health.

The mighty increase in the number and size of our medical schools that occurred in the past quarter-century, especially in the past fifteen years, took place because of the generally perceived national need for a substantial increase in the number of physicians. At the same time, the growing development of new knowledge and the explosion in technology, centered in the medical schools, resulted in the assumption by clinical faculties of the responsibility for a greater proportion of the diagnosis and treatment of complex problems known as tertiary care (for example, open heart surgery, organ transplants, burn centers, brain surgery). They now clearly dominate this crucial element of medical care where the "medical miracle" is now commonly expected. These developments, coupled with the intimate involvement of the teaching programs for medical students and residents with tertiary care and the increased number of hospitals affiliated with medical schools, have given these schools a pervasive and dominant influence on the future shape, content, quality, and cost of medical services to the public. Much more than any other professional school in a university, medical schools and their associated teaching hospitals set the pattern of practice for the future, not only through their teaching per se, but also because their faculties exercise increasing control over a growing and vital portion of medical care.

THE HOSPITAL: FROM PERIPHERY TO CENTER

Our nation's hospitals have also undergone dramatic and radical change in this century. Starting out as places "on the other side of the hill" for the poor,—essentially undifferentiated social institutions that primarily provided shelter—they have been transformed as knowledge relevant to disease became available. With the discovery of anesthesia and the value of aseptic techniques, surgery became safer. Because of the teamwork and equipment needed, surgery was done in hospitals. Critically ill patients began to be admitted so they could obtain the continuous nursing and medical care they needed. As laboratory medicine developed, patients with medical (rather than surgical) problems were admitted to hospitals even if not critically ill, in order to take advantage of those services. This was followed, in the second quarter of this century, by a trend to admit pregnant women to hospitals for the delivery of their children—to increase the safety of this physiological, nondisease process for both the mother and child, through the use of equipment and services that could not be provided for deliveries at home. Later, with the burgeoning of laboratory tests and radiological and other diagnostic procedures, hospitals, especially the larger ones, were increasingly used as diagnostic and referral centers.

Once a place to which patient's were sent to linger, to die, or at most to have surgery, the hospital became essential to the conduct of the practice of most physicians. In virtually all specialties, including general practice or family medicine, at least a few of the physician's patients would be in the hospital at all times, looked after either by the referring physician, consultants or residents. In deciding where to practice, physicians looked for the ready availability of a hospital. Communities of moderate or even small size came to believe that they should have their own hospital; it was seen as an essential community resource, much like a school system or a well-equipped fire department. For this reason the funding of general hospital development in this century (both capital costs and operating deficits) has fallen primarily to communities, voluntary associations or local government.

General hospitals in the United States began to develop in colonial times. The first general hospital, the Pennsylvania Hospital in Philadelphia, was opened in 1751. It was not until a quarter-century later, in 1775, that the second, the New York Hospital, was opened. A survey done in 1873 identified only 178 hospitals. Concentrated in five states (53 of them in New York alone), they were predominantly of the poorhouse type. In the 1880s hospitals began to add operating rooms designed for asepsis. The first hospital in the United States to establish a laboratory of bacteriology and chemistry for use in diagnosis and treatment was the Lankenau Hospital in Philadelphia in 1889. When medical specialties, beyond general medicine and surgery, began to develop, hospitals were crucial to their practice. These developments, together with the growth and rapid urbanization of the nation's population, were responsible for a dramatic increase in the number of hospitals thereafter. By 1909, there were 4359 hospitals of all types with a total bed capacity of 421,000.[16]

Though the community general hospital, most usually under voluntary auspices, became the dominant institution, other specialized hospitals developed to meet the needs of children, women, patients with mental diseases, tuberculosis, and chronic orthopedic conditions, and other specific problems. As the community hospitals—nonfederal short-term general and certain special hospitals—grew in number, they assumed a major and controlling role in medical care.

By 1938, the number of hospitals of all types reached 6166, bringing their total bed capacity to 1,161,380. Thus, there was an increase of 270 percent in total beds in three decades.[17] The Hospital Survey and Construction Act of 1946, commonly called the Hill-Burton Act, made federal funds available for the construction of hospital facilities according to state plans. The greatest increase in such beds occurred in the 1960s, when Hill-Burton funds were most freely available. Nationwide, the availability of community hospital beds rose from 3.2 per thousand persons in 1940 to 4.6 per thousand in 1975, where is has since remained.[18] In 1976, short-term general hospitals represented 87 percent of the country's 7271 hospitals of all types. With a capacity of over one million beds, these 6361 hospitals ranged widely in size. Out of 6009 nonfederal general medical and specialty hospitals, for example, 1519 (25.2 percent) had fewer than fifty beds. These small institutions are limited by their size in their capability to provide complex care. They can provide only relatively simple care and therefore can meet only part of their community's need for hospitalization. There were

1635 hospitals with 200 or more beds, 27.2 percent of the total. Only 305, 5 percent, had 500 beds or more. Hospitals with 200 or more beds, however, represented almost two-thirds (62 percent) of total bed capacity.[19] Thus the larger hospitals dominate in terms of their share of beds nationally, as well as in the broader range of services they can provide.

Utilization of these hospitals has changed significantly; the proportion of the population hospitalized has increased but the average duration of their stay in the hospital has declined. These changes became evident in the second quarter of this century. In a study at the Beth Israel Hospital in Boston, for example, it was found that nineteen patients per bed were admitted in 1932, compared with thirty-two in 1952.[20] This trend has continued. Nationally, in 1950, 110 persons per thousand population were admitted to all general and special hospitals excluding psychiatric and tuberculosis. The average length of stay was 10.6 days. By 1974, however, the rate of patients admission had increased by 50 percent to 165 per thousand and the average length of stay had fallen by 20 percent to 8.7 days. By 1977 it had fallen to 8.3 days.[21]

The trends in hospital costs in the same period are also enlightening. In 1950 total expense in community hospitals was $16 per patient day. It rose to $128 in 1974 and to $198 by 1977. During much of this period, and since then, the rate of increase of hospital costs has been much higher than the rise in general inflation.[22] One important element in the increase in costs is the continuous increase in the number of employees in hospitals. In community hospitals nationwide, the number of full-time-equivalent employees per hundred average daily patients rose from 226 in 1960 to 369 in 1977, an average annual increase of just under 3 percent.[23] This growth was largely due to the additional tasks performed in these institutions as the range and complexity of diagnosis and treatment procedures increased. Hospital care expenditures in the nation have, for quite some time now, claimed the largest share of the health care dollar, rising from $3.9 billion (30.4 percent of total expenditures) in 1950 to $76 billion (39.5 percent) in 1979, an average annual increase of 11.2 percent.[24] For the year ending March 1980, hospital expenditures reached $88.5 billion, representing 40.3 percent of national health care expenditures. The increase in hospital expenditures for the year was 13.5 percent.[25]

A notable trend in recent decades has been the growing use of hospital facilities for ambulatory care. Ambulatory cases are those in which the patient travels to the site of care and leaves it the same day; by far the greatest number of such visits are made to the outpatient departments and emergency rooms of hospitals. From small beginnings at the turn of the century, the rate of growth in the utilization of the hospital for ambulatory care rose steadily until the 1950s, after which the rise became much steeper. The total number of such visits to all hospitals in 1975 was 256,067,000, for an average annual rate of 1202 visits per thousand people. Almost 80 percent of these were visits to nonfederal general hospitals. Of these, 34.3 percent were made to the hospital emergency rooms, a rate of 327.2 visits per thousand persons.[26] This type of care, providing services generally not otherwise available, constitutes an increasingly significant element of the services provided by many hospitals. Not only is the hospital the locus of care for virtually all emergencies, but the public has come to expect it to provide medical care on a twenty-four hour basis for those who are unable to obtain such care from a local physician at the time they perceive the need for it. The hospital became the family physician for many people, especially those in the city ghetto areas.

The care now provided by the larger hospitals encompasses a widening series of specialties beyond general medicine, general surgery, and obstetrics, including medical and surgical subspecialties, psychiatric care, premature nursery, neonatal intensive care, burn care, open heart surgery, occupational therapy, and CAT scanning, to mention just a few. The special facilities and specialized medical and allied personnel needed for such services and the increased resource costs have produced a differentiation of hospitals into various levels of comprehensiveness which depend significantly, though not solely, upon the size of the hospital. The most comprehensive is one which has the facilities and the appropriately qualified staff to perform the most complex patient care that is known in the tertiary hospital. The principle of hospital regionalization emerged in response to the development of very large, comprehensive tertiary-care institutions. The Hill-Burton Act of 1946 required that statewide hospital plans be developed which incorporated the principle of state-wide planning and encouraged voluntary areawide planning. Such planning for the size and function of individual hospitals was to follow the logical principle of differentiating the range of services undertaken by the smaller institutions and by the largest and most comprehensive ones, now known as tertiary-care institutions.[27] This requirement was observed only in the most general sense. Over the past two decades, the rapid growth of new technology applicable to medical care, has again highlighted the need for the regionalization approach. Health Systems Agencies, set up in the past decade, have focused most of their efforts on the appropriate number and location of such facilities and services to achieve the twin goals of cost containment and good quality.

All states except Ohio require that hospitals be licensed, but the requirements and standards for such licensure vary considerably from state to state. After World War II, a national voluntary accreditation program was launched by a special organization set up for this purpose, the Joint Commission on Accreditation of Hospitals. As of January 1976, approximately 5000 hospitals were accredited by this body. Such accreditation has become a requirement for eligibility for payment by such major payers as Blue Cross, Medicare, and Medicaid.

Starting out as a facility peripheral to the day-to-day medical care of a population, the community hospital has become the control point of our medical care system. The nature of its work has been greatly intensified both for the care of acutely ill patients and for the diagnosis and treatment of others. Scientific progress, rapidly expanding technology, and the increasing specialization of practitioners and allied health personnel have produced a profound differentiation in the scope of services provided by hospitals of different sizes, location, and types. The larger hospitals generally offer a wider scope of patient treatment and carry out functions unique to them. An increasing number of these hospitals are also vital to the education of a growing number of different types of health personnel and to medical research. In the past decade, the organized involvement of hospitals in the education of health personnel, while concentrated in the largest general hospitals, has begun to include somewhat smaller community general hospitals and specialized institutions. The development of the area health education centers in twenty states illustrates this movement well.

THE ACADEMIC MEDICAL CENTER EMERGES

This review of the growth and profound changes in medical education and in hospitals during the twentieth century helps us understand the current status and complexities of the academic medical center. Emerging from a revolution in medical education and the scope of hospital services, it has become the apex of the hospital and medical care system. As medical schools have extended and deepened their day-to-day relationships with the hospitals they own, or with which they are affiliated, difficult issues of purpose, control, and financing have emerged—problems for which easy or widely satisfactory solutions have not been readily available.

At the same time as our academic medical centers have assumed the leading role in shaping the content and effectiveness of medical care, and in fact are providing a significant portion of it, the public interest in making medical care of acceptable quality available to everyone, regardless of place of residence or social station, has become a basic tenet of our nation's avowed public policy. This, too, has produced difficult issues of purpose, control, and financing for the academic medical centers—problems for which generally suitable solutions have yet to be developed. The vexing questions facing these centers, while not entirely new, are today strong and persistent. They arise from the interaction between public policy, which encouraged their growth, and the inherent nature of the academic medical centers as they have evolved. Certain basic elements of their structure and function constitute the nexus of the dilemmas they face internally (as between the affiliated hospitals and the medical school and between the medical school and the university) and externally (among the academic medical center, the relevant government agencies, and the community and region served).

Medical schools are either public, supported by and responsible to state governments, or privately supported under the aegis of a university board (elected or appointed, sometimes self-appointed). In 1962, there were 40 public schools and 45 privately sponsored schools. Almost all of the many new schools set up since then have been sponsored by state governments. By 1977-1978, there were 124 accredited schools in operation. State governments had started 34 new schools and 5 were privately sponsored.

One prominent difference between public or private sponsorship is in the degree and immediacy of public accountability. Clearly a private university trustee board which has the final responsibility for policy and financing of its medical school, as dedicated, knowledgeable, and farsighted as it may be, is generally not as directly concerned about public needs and perceptions, particularly in the state and region, as a state university board or the state legislature is likely to be. This difference, while still present, has been sharply reduced in the past two decades, largely because of the heavy investment of tax funds in the support of medical schools. The proportion of medical school revenues from the federal government has dropped from a level of over 50 percent in the late 1960s, but continues to be substantial, between 25 and 30 percent.[28]

In addition, especially in the 1970s, a number of state governments began to provide subsidies to private medical schools in their state, generally on a per capita basis in relation to the total number or to the increase in the number of in-state students admitted. For the school year 1978-1979, thirty-five of the nation's fifty-one private medical schools received $79 million from the sixteen states in which they are located. In two states, Ohio and Texas, the level of state support was equal to the state appropriation for medical students to the public schools of the state. In the other states the amount was fixed and below the level appropriated to the state schools.[29]

A typical example of this type of state aid is the North Carolina program of "Private Medical School Aid," which has been in operation since 1969.

This program is designed to encourage the Bowman Gray School of Medicine and the Duke University School of Medicine, through contractual agreements with the Board of Governors, to expand medical education opportunities for citizens of the State through enrolling increased numbers of North Carolinians, to provide funds for financial aid to needy North Carolina students enrolled in these schools: and thereby to increase the supply of physicians. The Board of Governors pays capitation grants to the two medical schools for each North Carolina resident enrolled as a full-time student studying for the M.D. degree.[30]

The capitation payment for Bowman Gray Medical School, for example, is now $8000 per student, of which $1000 is put in the scholarship pool, the remainder in an unrestricted pool. The encouragement which the state of North Carolina hoped for indeed took place. By 1973 the school undertook to increase the enrollment of state residents in each entering class to forty-five; three years later, it agreed to raise this figure again, to sixty-five, or 60 percent of the class. On this basis this school received a total of $1,813,000 in the academic year 1979-1980. This amount represents 3.9 percent of this school's total expenditure for that year.[31] Thus Bowman Gray, like many other private institutions nationwide, has assumed a more public posture which tends to blur the difference between public and private schools with respect to public accountability.

As we have pointed out, all schools find themselves deeply dependent upon federal policies and programs which affect their sources and amounts of support. But in addition, two-thirds of the private schools in the nation are also receiving sizable funds from their state government, thus distinctly linking them with its health and higher education policies. Although their linkage and dependence may not be as great as that of the state-owned schools, because the amount of money they receive is smaller, the dependence is as great as the value of the state subsidy to each school—usually not inconsiderable. Thus all schools, public and private, must take state and federal public policy into account as they conduct their programs and plan for the future. Certainly, there have always been a few voices in medical schools urging that more overt and organized attention be given by their institutions to the immediate and long-term needs of their region and the nation. The great increase in the importance of tax funds in support of medical schools helps to strengthen these voices at least a little.

The medical faculty has unique problems in carrying out its multiple functions in this framework within its larger university family. Teaching and research are readily understood by their colleagues in other fields of learning and by the trustees, but they do present some special problems. For example, the medical school research budget is generally the largest in the university. The faculty-student ratio is by far the highest. Consequently, the medical faculty spends far more money than the other professional schools, the social sciences, the humanities, or the arts. In some large universities the medical faculty's share amounts to 25 percent or more of the total. In one relatively small university, it is 60 percent. But the most distinctive activity of the medical faculty is its deep involvement, often on or adjacent to the university campus, in the continuous delivery of medical care. The rest of the university does not share such responsibilities (with the exception, to a much smaller degree, of some of the other health profession schools). At the same time, these medical care activities are the most predominant and the most prestigious in the public eye.

Large size, public prestige, relatively massive expenditures, high salaries, extensive service activities, and increasing public interest and attention characterize the medical schools as unique insitutions in our universities. The result is intrauniversity tension and a sense, shared by the medical faculty, the university administration, and the trustees, that the presence of the school in the university is a mixed blessing. The medical faculty, while believing sincerely that its activities constitute university functions in the best meaning of the term, often find that the usual, hallowed, and time-tested standards and procedures of the university simply do not meet their needs as they see them. Hence they insist upon and generally get separate treatment which, while probably necessary, does not endear them to their sister units and faculties. An eminent academic leader, asked why he left a top administrative position at a leading university for a similar position in a university of distinctly lesser reputation, explained, "It's my home state and, besides, it doesn't have a medical school." Conversely, deans of medical schools and their department chairmen often complain, "The university administration simply does not understand us!"

HOSPITAL-MEDICAL SCHOOL RELATIONSHIPS

Special problems are created by the relationship of the medical faculty with its teaching hospital or hospitals. Traditionally and most commonly, there is one major hospital among the hospitals with which the school has its primary affiliation. In 1979, there were sixty-three university-owned hospitals, more of them in state than in private universities. Hospital ownership and operation represents an increasingly complex and high-cost service program that generates administrative problems and demands strikingly different from the university's accustomed scope of academic activities and procedures. When the university does not own the teaching hospital, it still has to face unaccustomed problems of purpose, control, and financing which are inherent in the intimate working relationship of its medical faculty with a complex service facility and patient care program.

The hospitals involved with medical school educational programs are not all of a single type. Nor are the scope and size of their educational program or the nature of their relationship with the medical school always the same. The most comprehensive study of the affiliations and working relationships between hospitals and medical schools, by Sheps et al., was published in 1965.[32] The general topography of these affiliations has remained the same since that time, although some changes of course, have accompanied the large increase in the number of medical schools and the size of their student bodies, and the rising interest in primary care. As reported and defined by medical schools in 1962, roughly half the affiliations were of a major nature and the rest minor.[33] In 1979 the Council of Teaching Hospitals of the Association of American Medical Colleges (AAMC) classified teaching hospitals into three groups.

> The first group includes hospitals which regard their service and educational missions as inseparable, first-order objectives. Neither mission is subordinate to the other when the institution defines its role or plans its future. A second group of hospitals at the other extreme includes those which view their educational mission as a distinct and separable addition to their patient care mission. These hospitals are primarily concerned with the impact of educational programs on the quality of care and institutional prestige; clinical education is clearly viewed as an accessory or option which could be deleted if necessary. The final category, the middle group, includes hospitals which are less clear about the relationship between their teaching and service missions. In many cases, these hospitals wish to be viewed by the public as being in the first category, but they still separate the patient care and education components of institutional decision making.[34]

This classification framework really represents a continuum, along which the precise location of a given hospital must be very much a matter of judgment. More significantly, the AAMC statement embodies an assumption about the separability and equality of missions which merits examination—a bit later in this chapter. The context and organization of the education programs carried out in hospitals, and their impact upon the organization and control of patient care, shape the day-by-day activities of these hospitals and reflect the depth, strength, and pervasiveness of the affiliation. A critical factor is the types of learners who come to the institution—medical students, residents or others: how many, for how long, and in what special fields of practice? The most deeply involved teaching hospitals are those that make continuous arrangements for the education of both medical students and residents in all major clinical fields: medicine, surgery, pediatrics, obstetrics/gynecology, and psychiatry. Our estimate is that this classical situation is found in only about one-third of the affiliated hospitals. Some hospitals have a residency program only. Others will only provide a short-term experience from time to time for a selected number of medical students in one particular field. And there are many other combinations.

The number of affiliations for a medical school is not uniform. It varies as does the scope of the affiliations. In 1962 the median number of affiliations for public medical schools was five; for private schools it was seven. The overall mean was six.[35] Since then the overall mean, for all types of affiliations, has increased to about ten. The great growth in demand for educational opportunities within the framework of medical care delivery is evidenced by doubling of medical student enrollment from 30,288 in 1960 to 60,455 in 1977, accompanied by a more than fourfold growth in the number of full-time clinical faculty from 7201 to 33,059.[36]

The implications of a teaching affilition for a hospital will vary in terms of its authority and responsibility for policy and planning and for the range and employment of selected medical staff. Staffing for twenty-four-hour in-house services coverage and financing will vary widely depending upon the scope and comprehensiveness of its educational obligations balanced against the needs of its patient care programs. The hospitals most influenced by affiliation are those whose entire range of service is involved in teaching programs at both the medical student and resident level; about one-third of affiliated institutions fall in this group. Generally, each medical school will have at least one core hospital, sometimes two and less often three, which is a general hospital with teaching programs for medical students and residency programs in at least four major services: medicine, surgery, obstetrics/gynecology, and pediatrics. Although affiliation with a medical school influences the provision of services in each hospital, the largest and most pervasive influence is seen in the core hospitals.

Because of the variation in the practical meaning of an affiliation with a medical school, and in the ways this is reported by the hospitals themselves, the AMA, and the AAMC, it is difficult to be precise about the scope of such arrangements in different hospitals or the number and types of institutions involved. Overall, however, there are now approximately 1000 hospitals with some type of affilition involving programmed education activities.[37] This, then, is the wide orbit within which our medical schools function and exercise influence, if not control. Of these, 792 are community short-term general and other special hospitals. Affiliated hospitals constitute only 13.3 percent of this class, but tend to be among the larger institutions. Because of their size, they account for 40 percent of the total beds and provide care for 30 percent of the outpatient and emergency visits made by people seeking help at community hospitals. All types of affiliated institutions are now spending over $35 billion, at least 40 percent of the total spent by all the hospitals in these categories including those that do not have any medical school affiliation.[38]

As noted earlier, the strength and depth of the affiliation and its effect upon the nature of the patient care depends upon the scope and character of the education program and the degree of control exercised by the medical faculty upon the hospital's facilities and the conduct of its clinical services. Although core hospitals are generally similar in their basic interactions with their medical schools, the closeness of the union varies in terms of its formal structure and the locus of control.

The best approximation available of the number and types of core teaching hospitals is found in the membership of the Council of Teaching Hospitals (COTH), a voluntary membership unit of the Association of American Medical Colleges. In 1977 COTH had 402 members with medical school affiliations, most of which were of a major nature. Of these, 63 are university owned, 44 are state owned, and 41 are county or city owned. By far the largest number, 241, are community voluntary institutions, of which 41 are church related. Though they range in size, most of them are quite large—73 percent having 411 beds or more and 22 percent having 746 beds or more. Though the 323 short-term nonfederal hospitals in COTH which reported in 1977 constituted only 5.4 percent of all such hospitals in the United States, they represented 18.4 percent of the beds, 20.4 percent of all admissions, 31.3 percent of the outpatient visits, 30.3 percent of total payroll, and 27.9 percent of total expenditures. They also had over half the employed physicians in terms of full-time equivalents, 70 percent of the interns and residents, and 26.9 percent of total personnel. The latter proportion had increased by more than 75 percent since 1973.

Other comparisons between 1973 and 1977 are also instructive. The average cost per admission rose 84 percent, to $2383, in these COTH hospitals, while it rose only 52 percent to $1509, in the others.[39] The higher costs of these hospitals are presumably due to their treatment of a disproportionate number of complex cases and the cost of education. In 1979, the four core teaching hospitals affiliated with North Carolina's four medical schools accounted for 20 percent of the state's hospital expenditures, though only 10.6 percent of its nonfederal general hospital beds.[40] As would be expected because of their medical school affiliation and large average size, the COTH member institutions provide a high proportion of specialized services in the nation. Representing just under 7 percent of the country's hospitals, COTH institutions constitute 59.7 percent of those providing genetic counseling services, 51 percent of the burn care units, and 39.5 percent of the open heart surgery units, to name only a few such services.[41]

Most new developments in patient care are first explored and instituted in the teaching hospitals, in part because of the presence of full-time faculty members doing research in clinical fields and in part because of the volume of patients available in the larger hospitals, especially those with a substantial role as a referral center (often a corollary, if not a condition, of affiliation). The extent to which useful new services or modalities of care are then made available in non-teaching hospitals depends upon such factors as the expected frequency of patients needing such care, the size of the hospital, the cost of equipment and facilities, and the need and availability of highly specialized professional and technical personnel. With few exceptions, however, the academic medical center is now the place where changes in the nature, scope, and cost of care are first implemented, if not originally developed.

Many of these medical centers now have annual operating budgets for the medical school and one major teaching hospital of well over $100 million, with a few now exceeding $200 million.[42] They have come to occupy the salient controlling position in the education and training of doctors and an increasing number of other health professionals and technologists for work in our medical care system. The size and range of this increase is far beyond that represented by the increase in the number of medical schools alone. In the fifteen-year period from 1962-1963 to 1977-1978, the number of interns and residents in programs under medical school auspices increased by 120 percent to over 38,000. The number of graduate students in the biomedical sciences and in other fields related to medicine tripled to over 15,000 and all other students in these schools increased over threefold to 40,000. Thus in 1977-1978 the teaching responsibilities of medical faculties nationwide extended to over 154,000 students of various types. Of these 60,456 were medical students and 38,783 were interns or residents.[43]

Most of the health-related research in the United States is carried out by members of the medical faculties. These same faculties are responsible for the staffing and operation of their tertiary-care referral teaching hospitals—institutions that set the pace and the pattern for what is considered to be good-quality practice for the nation as a whole.

As a rule, the academic medical center serves as the central base of a medical school's activities. But some exceptions to this pattern have developed since the middle of the 1960s, when an unprecedented increase in the establishment of new medical schools began. Some of these were unable or unwilling to establish their organizational base in the classical fashion, that is, the academic medical center with a major hospital as a tertiary-care referral center which the university owns or whose patient care the medical school otherwise controls. Although these schools are in universities, they describe themselves as "community based" because their educational approach rests largely upon using the patient care framework of community hospitals rather than the tertiary-care hospital staffed or controlled by full-time medical faculty. The leading and oldest example of such a school is the College of Human Medicine of Michigan State University at Lansing. There are some eighteen such schools at present and more will be said about them later.

PROGRAM GOALS—BALANCE OR CONFLICT?

The academic medical center, a peculiarly American entity, has become a very large, complex set of related operations. The goals of these centers are customarily stated as education, research, and patient care. However, this simplistic formulation can be misleading, as A. W. Snoke and a few others have pointed out. In 1960, Snoke delineated the inherent problem in a pithy discussion of the issues that arise between the medical school and the hospital. He presented the problem of combining these three functions in a manner that would satisfy the needs of students, teachers, researchers, and patients—in the context of the hospital as a community institution and the community as a whole.

In an attempt to find a title that might be as descriptive but somewhat more provocative, three other possibilities came to mind.
1. The Teaching Hospital—A Study in Institutional Schizophrenia
2. The Teaching Hospital—A Philosophical Paradox
3. The Teaching Hospital—A Tipsy Tripod[44]

Snoke's formulation of the issues has very slowly gained some acceptance. Furthermore, recognition is slowly developing that a fourth goal must be added to the traditional trinity of education, research, and patient care. In their 1965 study, Sheps et al. recommended that a new goal be recognized and attended to.

> The suggestion is therefore made that a fourth goal be added to provide greater understanding and stability: the goal of community service. This is viewed as being different from, and larger than, patient care. Patient care, in terms of medical care for the individual is, of course, a form of community service. Research and education also are forms of community service.
>
> The study group conceives of the goal of community service in a somewhat different context than patient care, the latter being aimed at the individual patient in a relatively narrow sense. By community service is meant a willingness on the part of the teaching hospital (and the faculty of the affiliated medical school) to take its proper place in the whole range of health services needed in the community. It is intended to mean what has often been called 'readiness to serve.'. . . It may mean operating a unit for alcoholics . . . operating a unit for long term care, affiliating with a nursing home, taking part in a home care program, or many other possibilities.
>
> Although it is understandable, and oftentimes even desirable for the individual professor to be single-minded and dedicated to his research and teaching, it is the study group's opinion that it is most regrettable, if not unforgivable, for hospitals affiliated with medical schools to be less than fully aware of their broad responsibilities towards the goal of community service. Where a teaching hospital is actively making efforts to pursue the goal of community service, it follows that the medical school with which it is affiliated must be ready to share these efforts wholeheartedly.[45]

With a few noteworthy exceptions, most medical schools in the mid-1960s did not believe that community service per se constituted an important objective for them. Today, it is an obligation which we believe they cannot escape, as unwelcome as this fact may sometimes be. The new community-based medical schools have made a clear commitment to carry out their academic obligations in the context of community service. Among the older, well-established, prestigious, and more traditional academic medical centers, a number have begun to think seriously about facing this challenge. Most have done so with a good bit of anguish and uncertainty mixed with some regret that the "good old days" seem to have been vanished.

As seen within the academic medical centers, the problem of determining and achieving the appropriate balance between the four goals of education, research, patient care, and community service is a difficult and trying task. The traditional three goals are often reiterated with the implication not only that they are interrelated and that efforts toward one always help the others, but that the problem of emphasis does not exist. This is not the case however. First, it is unrealistic to assume that all clinical faculty members are *equally* interested in, and committed to, teaching, research, and patient care. Nor should this be expected. The ultimate balance is also influenced by the availability of resources directed at each of these three goals. Thus the overall institutional program reflects the mix or balance of those interests and opportunities and the time and effort devoted to them.

The problems of providing community service are especially troublesome to most medical faculty members and produce tensions within the academic medical center. On the one hand, this goal is one that all hospitals have long realized they must address. More recently, medical schools have had to acknowledge this obligation, even though many take the view that community service issues are not of their making and are more properly left to society and the medical profession as a whole to resolve. Although few centers will now risk openly disclaiming the goal of community service, for many of them it arouses little interest. They tend to do as much as seems necessary but as little as possible, because they sincerely believe that the community service effort deflects them from their more important and traditional responsibilities. On the other hand, some centers openly avow the committment and are carrying it out with increasing effectiveness.

Most academic medical centers would agree with the Council of Teaching Hospitals that "their service and education missions [are] inseparable, first-order objectives."[46] More open to question is the COTH assertion that "neither mission is subordinate to the other when the institution defines its role or plans for its future." There is no doubt that these objectives are interrelated and interdependent and that each facilitates the other in crucial and indispensable ways. They are not, however, inseparable. They are separate goals which do not, in fact, always each reinforce the other.

Certain types of educational and research activities can, if not carefully monitored and controlled from the point of view of patient care, result in poor service performance. Similarly, when patient care is poor because appropriate facilities and staff are lacking, education suffers as well. Furthermore, the developments of recent years have made it more compelling than ever before that hospitals look carefully to their communitywide responsibilities. With the decline in the role of philanthropic payment for medical care, the great expansion of organized third-party payment, both voluntary and governmental, and the emergence of the teaching hospital as a large, leading site for primary care as well as highly specialized health services, the public's expectations of these institutions have grown in strength and cogency and cannot be disregarded or readily turned in other directions. Moreover, the current surplus of hospital beds in many communities has produced a new competitive situation for many hospitals, potentially threatening their financial solvency.

Thus, the teaching hospital, like other hospitals, is today acutely conscious of an overt, rather than secondary, goal of community service. It will, of course, always be ready to make accommodations to its education function, but it is finding it increasingly difficult to subordinate its service responsibilities to these purposes. Until recently, the medical schools, focus on the training of clinical experts in increasingly specialized fields has emphasized inpatient care and has influenced the selection of patients for admission to the hospital. It has also minimized interest in preventive aspects of medical care and in posthospital care services. At the small risk of oversimplification, the issue is whether the faculty will give up the right to select "interesting" and "appropriate" patients and instead provide professional care for patients with a much wider spectrum of problems. The centers are beginning to realize that they cannot retain the recent past just as it has been, and that they cannot long stave off the fundamental issues. The exclusion of, or discrimination against, certain types of health problems in the area serviced by the hospital creates problems for it. It is not surprising, therefore, that the issues of community service and financial viability of the affiliated hospital are now the subject of much anguished and exasperating discussion in many academic medical centers.

Given the great growth of productive research in medical schools of the past quarter-century and the consequent overriding emphasis upon research performance as the foundation of medical education and the major basis for the appointment and promotion of faculty, it is not surprising that most schools give the greatest emphasis to the research goal. Continued growth of the research activities of an academic medical center has come to be expected. The onset of a steady state of financing for research (or at best a greatly reduced rate of escalation) has produced much concern and dismay, accompanied by a search for other sources of research support and intense, perhaps jealous, questioning of the commitment of resources for other goals in the academic medical center.

With their educational efforts too, new problems have arisen which highlight the issues of relevance and balance within the centers. Having responded to the national demand of the past fifteen years for more physicians and related personnel by greatly expanding their student body, in some cases doubling it, the academic medical centers now find the federal government warning of a "doctor glut" and withdrawing its financial support for teaching programs per se. In addition, state governments and Congress have indicated clearly, by their additional financial support for selected educational purposes, their belief that the centers have grossly neglected the preparation of physicians for primary care and are training too many specialists of certain types. This issue requires attention as decisions are made about the number of physicians for different types of specialties each academic medical center should undertake to train in the next decade. Understandably, this type of reappraisal is difficult and agonizing for the leaders and faculty members who have helped bring their centers to their present form, size, and areas of emphasis.

In this period of economic restraint and greater accountability to the public, the task of allocating effort and financial resources among the four goals of the academic medical center inevitably provokes much discussion and some conflict. This conflict is useful because it highlights the basic elements of activity that need to be brought into balance—a new balance—for most centers. In striving for that balance, it helps to realize that the goals cannot be substituted for each other, and that each should be seen simultaneously as an end and a means. The community and the hospital see patient care and community service as ends in themselves. The medical schools see them as means for education and research. On the other hand, education is seen by the hospital and the community as a means for improving and ensuring a high level of health care performance. Research is seen not only as an end in itself but also as a means toward improving the atmosphere for learning and making the latest knowledge readily available for application on behalf of patients.

This struggle for a new balance among the diverse goals and efforts of the academic medical center does not take place in a vacuum. Indeed, it is particularly discomfiting to the leaders of the centers and their colleagues that their decisions about these issues do not remain in their own enclave. Because they are expected to meet publicly expressed social needs, their policy decisions are subject to open scrutiny. Not since the public discussion in their communities of the medical schools criticized by Flexner in 1910 has there been such public attention to medical schools in this country. Perhaps this signals the end of the Flexnerian era, ushering in a new one with a transcending, and thus unifying, societal purpose.

These problems produce tension and conflict not only within the academic medical center and the university, but also between it and strong forces external to it. From the point of view of state and national policy, the academic medical centers have four pervasive major responsibilities: the preparation of sufficient medical manpower in the various specialties including primary care; the conduct of research relevant to health and disease; the delivery of health services in appropriate functional coordination with other medical resources in their community and region; and shaping the pattern and costs of care in the future. The four medical center goals described earlier must be implemented so as to meet these societal needs and expectations. In some particular respects, the public expectations may be somewhat simplistic; nevertheless the centers have vital contributions to make in achieving each of these goals and would be unwise to remain aloof from them.

As with all new and disturbing ideas, a new role for these centers was suggested by a few farsighted leaders in medical education long before the notion could command anything more than polite attention from their colleagues. For example, George P. Berry wrote in 1958, while he was dean of the Harvard Medical School:

> The medical schools are the wellsprings whence will flow the better health of tomorrow. They must constantly adjust their educational offerings for future doctors to the changing conditions and needs of society . . . students must learn about the factors that affect the availability and quality of medical care. They need to learn also how to evaluate their experiences and those of others in a number of developing programs such as, for example, health insurance and a group practice. Good medicine cannot be practiced independently of the intricate framework in which other health personnel function. The clinical medicine of the future will be indissolubly a part of the future organization of medical service with all the relevant professional activities, facilities and financing.[47]

The historical development of the academic medical center explains the dilemmas it faces and its difficulties in confronting this issue squarely and deciding upon the changes needed. The changes recommended above need not necessarily prejudice the opportunities for these centers to carry out their research and teaching functions effectively. They may even be strengthened, in new ways. Few centers, thus far, have been able to overcome their difficulties in making these decisions. Instead, there is much puzzlement, wringing of hands, and some resentment. They feel unappreciated and beleaguered. They are described, aptly, as "A Stressed American Institution" in a paper by D. E. Rogers and R. J. Blendon of the Robert Wood Johnson Foundation.[48] The authors set forth a number of problems which they believe have produced this stress. The most significant of these are:

1. *Problems posed by their interface with the public.* Various develop-ments have made the centers a big business and greatly enlarged their role in delivering and shaping medical care.

2. *The problem of the location of many centers.* One-quarter of these centers are located in the central decaying areas of large cities, areas deemed undesirable and dangerous by those who live else-where. The poor of these ghettos represent an increasing propor-tion of the patients coming to these centers for care. Physicians did not find these deteriorating areas desirable practice sites, thus in-creasing the number of people who have no alternative but to turn to the centers for virtually all their care. "There was a falling off in referrals of patients of higher incomes to the academic medical centers. Thus, the centers were left with vastly more patients than they could adequately manage, many of them unable to pay for the services they needed, inexorably rising costs of the whole aca-demic enterprise and a rapidly declining population of patients who had the kinds of complex problems teaching centers were best able to manage and who, because of resources, could also help foot the bill."

3. *Problems created by the current size of the academic medical centers.* The phenomenal growth of the medical school faculties and the number of personnel employed by the teaching hospitals has already been described. It is not uncommon for an academic medi-cal center to employ well over 5000 people, including faculty and supporting staff, hospital personnel, and residents. Added to this are the operational complexities and increased costs presented by the new technologies, which are generally first adopted by such centers and often concentrated there.

4. *With the implementation of Medicare and Medicaid, a large pro-portion of previously "charitable" medical care is now paid for by government funds.* In addition voluntary prepayment programs cover a large section of the population. Thus a great majority of hospital income, and a lesser but growing proportion of income earned by the clinical faculty comes from public or quasi-public agencies. These institutions demand accountability, in the form of various types of monitoring and complicated regulations. Thus the trend to public funding, while providing more certain sources and amounts of support, has made administration of the hospitals much more complex.

5. *The large size of the academic center, the large amount of money it spends, often well over $100 million, and the altered conditions*

under which much of these funds are provided, have produced unique new problems. Funds for research, teaching, and patient care, some of which were in the past often readily transferable to other related purposes, are now monitored more closely and need to be accounted for in terms of their specific purpose. Furthermore, centers can no longer independently determine their growth and emphasis, particularly in patient care, without overt and public reference to the needs of their community and region and its other medical resources. Formal requirements for such planning are now set forth by the federal government and carried out by the Health Systems Agency in each region.

NEW DIRECTIONS?

A new depth of understanding and special skills are needed for the planning and management of the academic medical center. Hospital administrators have received some training for this task in their professional education programs. Medical faculty members generally have no preparation for the skilled handling of such complexities.

The growth in types and size of activities is largely responsible for the increasing complexity of the policy, organizational, and day-to-day operational problems of the academic medical centers. These activities have become increasingly diverse and represent either basic interests generic to the medical faculty in its various parts or responses made by the faculty and its affiliated hospitals to patient care and community health needs. Public needs are now more strongly articulated through local, state, and federal governmental or quasi-governmental bodies. The latter control a widening range of policy and financing determinations which impinge or make demands upon elements of the center. While some of these public determinations provide great and relevant opportunities, they are often viewed within the centers as diversions, if not seriously damaging, from the traditional activities of the faculty. Thus, in recent years, there has been much discussion within the academic medical centers, in their universities, and in their national associations about the increasing outside pressures to which these centers are subjected. In sharp contrast to the cloistered atmosphere to which university faculties are accustomed, the centers are increasingly seen by the public and its representatives as *public* institutions— and are being treated that way.

The public's interest—and its great investment—in academic medical centers is an expression of its conviction that they constitute the crucial foundation for most efforts to achieve our national goal of making modern health services readily available to all our citizens. This has added new, competing pressures on the centers—pressures to which faculty are unaccustomed and which many faculty members and their leaders believe are irrelevant to their academic responsibilities. Deep differences in policy goals are apparent. Put simply, the conflict is between two quite different approaches to public policy for health. The one to which the academic medical centers are accustomed and are most comfortable with is the need to expand medical knowledge, medical technology, and specialization. This calls for more research with the expectation of more scientific and technological advances in knowledge, leading to improvement in diagnosis, treatment, and prevention. Public policy agrees with this approach and supports it quite well, but now expresses interest in the general scope and focus of the research and in expediting the application of new knowledge.

The other public policy approach, which has gathered strength steadily in the past fifteen years, is represented by the steps taken to implement the egalitarian social goal of making health services available to everyone and to do so as economically as possible consistent with providing services of good quality. As public programs toward this end take shape, the crucial role of the academic medical centers becomes clearer. They are indeed the wellsprings of the health care of the future. Their scope, size, and influence have so increased that the centers not only educate and train physicians and related personnel for professional and technical health services, but shape the future pattern and cost of health services through the range and volume of medical services they control and use as a framework for their educational programs.

Academic medical centers generally have not welcomed the demand that they correct the shortfall in physicians trained for primary care. Nor do they take readily to the notion that they should see to it that the number of people trained for each specialty approximates national and regional needs to avoid the surpluses that now obtain in certain fields, even though the centers, each in its own orbit, control the number of residency positions. Most of the centers believe that it is unreasonable to expect them to repair the deficit in the availability of physicians in the central cities and rural areas since the problem is not of their making. Yet in the public eye, it seems clear that the centers can and should make crucial contributions to solving these problems. In terms of the training and orientation of students, and research into and demonstrations of new approaches to the problems of access to medical care, the academic medical center can have a greater impact than virtually any other institutions or agencies.

During the past thirty years, as the academic medical centers have grown, they described themselves as national resources for health personnel and new knowledge and were seen and treated that way by federal public policy. In the past fifteen years, public policy has come to view them as vital elements in the solution of the national problems of access to good care and the control of its cost. This the centers did not bargain for. And with few exceptions, they are not prepared for their new role by either orientation or organization. Indeed, many think that they must be protected and insulated from such responsibilities because they will sully and depress the quality of their more traditional activities. This is the centers' predicament. Not only is public scrutiny directed to their traditional responsibilities in education and research, but demands are made in a completely new area: the centers are now charged with shaping the delivery and costs of medical care to the population to meet the twin goals of effectiveness and economy.

That these relatively new developments should produce surprise, dismay, concern, and frustration in academic medical centers is to be expected—given the way the centers developed, the manner in which decisions are made within them, and the great success they have had in carrying out the objectives they had earlier set for themselves. These traditional objectives have served very important societal functions. Now, however, public policy asks how this new knowledge, these new specialists, and this new technology should be deployed and organized to do the most good for the most people at the least cost. Most of the centers seem to believe that these are not questions they should be expected to address. Resolving these issues calls for work that is not only new, but very different. Why do that when there is so much more to be done in fields they are accustomed to working in? Furthermore, these new responsibilities involve close relationships with communities and a new set of agencies external to the university, whom they must trust as colleagues and partners and who are not under their direct purview. This represents a new experience, venturing into the unknown, and it is less controllable.

One rough measure of the mounting difficulties and frustrations produced by these pressures and problems of balance is the shortening tenure of medical school deans. In 1962, 65 percent of deans had served for five or more years, and there were only two acting deans. In 1974 only 22 percent had served for five years or more, and sixteen schools had acting deans. Over the period, the median tenure of deans had fallen from five to three years.[49] Data on the trend since then appear to indicate some improvement in this pattern. These complexities and the associated disenchantment are not limited to the dean's office. The pattern is also being seen now in the chairmanship of clinical departments; in medicine, for example, the median length of tenure is beginning to approach that of the deanship. Like deans, department heads must struggle to find the "right" balance among an ever widening series of research, educational, patient care, and community service activities funded from multiple sources; budgets may amount to several million dollars annually, with much of the funding unpredictable from year to year.

As Charles Dickens wrote, "It was the best of times. It was the worst of times." Certainly the road taken by our medical schools and hospitals since the Flexner report has brought brilliant and important successes in research, education, and practice. Now, after a period of great growth in size, research productivity, and prestige, the centers somehow appear to be not good enough. It is as though something went wrong on the way to the future. More is demanded of them. But not more of the same. Something different is expected—a much more direct relationship with community needs and social policy and the assumption by the centers of a set of direct responsibilities for the nature, effectiveness, and cost of the delivery of medical care itself. Except for the agricultural extension and research efforts of our land grant colleges, there is no precedent in the American university for this type of direct relationship with the public and immediate societal goals. Yet in the eyes of the public and its representatives, these expectations are not only reasonable but necessary. Academic medical centers are a vital national health resource and expect to be treated as such; they must be prepared to behave accordingly. They must expect, and welcome, not only public appreciation, adulation, and interest, but also public expectations, scrutiny and criticism.

Over the past fifteen years, the academic medical centers have become increasingly crucial to the achievement of public policy objectives in health for the population of the United States. At the same time, these centers have become increasingly dependent on public funds for the support of their traditional activities. Thus public policy and the academic medical centers are closely interdependent. One cannot succeed without the other. However, the tensions and conflicts that exist between them are deep and divisive. The institutions, agencies, and individuals leading each of these two sets of complex efforts need to understand each other better and to learn how to achieve their joint social ends much more directly. We believe that a much more effective partnership can be achieved, but not without substantial modifications of the goals of the centers and of the public policymaking framework of our nation. The goals of the centers can be appropriately balanced only by facing the fundamental issues of purpose, control, and financing—issues which need fresh attention in the public policy sphere as well as within the academic medical centers.

NOTES

1. Association of Academic Health Centers, *The Organization and Governance of Academic Health Centers.* Vol. 2, p. 12. Washington, D.C., April 1980.
2. A. Flexner, *On Medical Education in the United States and Canada.* Carnegie Fund for the Advancement of Education, Bulletin No. 4, p. 239.
3. *Ibid.*
4. *Ibid.,* p.x.
5. C. G. Sheps and C. Seipp, "The Medical School, Its Products and Its Problems," *Annals of American Association of Political Science,* Vol. 399, January 1972, p. 43.
6. Association of American Medical Colleges, *Medical Education: Institutions, Characteristics and Programs.* Washington, D. C., Aug. 1979, p. 17, Fig. 18; p. 21, Fig. 26.
7. *Ibid.,* p. 5; p. 17, Fig. 16.
8. "Medical Education in the United States 1975-76," *Journal of the American Medical Association,* Vol. 236 (Dec. 27, 1976), p. 2977. Cambridge Research Institute, *Trends Affecting the U.S. Health Care System.* Washington, D.C.: DHEW Publication No. HRA 76-14503.
9. Association of American Medical Colleges, *op. cit.,* p. 11.
10. U.S. Department of Health, Education and Welfare. (Public Health Service, 263), 1968. *Health Manpower Source Book,* Section 20: Manpower Supply and Educational Statistics for Selected Health Occupations, p. 19.
11. "Medical Education in the United States, 1979-80," *Journal of the American Medical Association,* Vol. 244, No. 25 (Dec. 26, 1980), p. 2820. See also Note 28 below.
12. "Medical Education in the United States, 1978-79," *Journal of the American Medical Association,* Vol. 243, No. 9 (Mar. 7, 1980), pp. 863-865.
13. Association of American Medical Colleges, *op. cit.,* p. 20, Fig. 25.
14. *Ibid.*
15. "State Funds in Support of Public and Private Medical Schools, 1979," *Journal of Medical Education,* Vol. 55, No. 10 (Oct. 1980), pp. 885-887.
16. R. A. Nelson, in J. Z. Bowers and E. F. Purcell (eds.), *Advances in American Medicine: Essays at the Bicentennial,* Vol. I. New York: Josiah Macy, Jr. Foundation, 1976, pp. 359 ff.
17. *Health Resource Statistics, Health Manpower and Health Facilities,* 1976-77 edition. Washington, D.C: U.S. Department of Health, Education and Welfare, p. 303.
18. *Health United States 1979.* Washington, D.C.: U.S. Department of Health, Eduction and Welfare, Pub. No. (PHS) 80-1232, p. 222.
19. *Health Resource Statistics,* p. 310, Table 207.
20. C. G. Sheps, "Hospitals and Clinical Teaching," *Journal of Medical Education,* Vol. 34, No. 10, p. 58.
21. *Statistical Abstract of the United States, 1979.* Washington, D.C.: U.S. Dept. of Commerce, p. 112, Table 174.
22. *Ibid.,* p. 111, Table 172.
23. *Health United States 1979,* p. 226.
24. *Ibid.,* p. 252.
25. *Health Care Financing Trends,* HCFA Office of Research, Demonstrations and Statistics, Vol. I, No. 4 (Summer 1980), pp. 1, 4.
26. *The Nation's Use of Health Resources, 1979.* Washington, D.C.: U.S. Department of Health, Education and Welfare, Pub. No. (PHS) 80-1420, p. 33.

27. C. G. Sheps and D. L. Madison, "The Medical Perspective," in E. Ginzberg, *Regionalization and Health Policy*. Washington, D.C.: U.S. Department of Health, Education and Welfare, DHEW Pub. No. (HRA) 77-623, pp. 15-22.
28. Association of American Medical Colleges, *op. cit.*, p. 21, Figure 26. See also Note 11 above.
29. "State Funds in Support of Public and Private Medical Schools," *op. cit.*, pp. 885-887.
30. Board of Governors of the University of North Carolina, *Budget Report*, 1979-81.
31. M. Meads, personal communication.
32. C. G. Sheps, P. A. Clark, J. W. Gerdes, E. Halpern, and N. Hershey, *Medical Schools and Hospitals: Interdependence for Education and Service*. Evanston: Association of American Medical Colleges, 1965. Also as Part Two, *Journal of Medical Education*, Vol. 40, (Sept. 1965).
33. *Ibid.*, p. 13.
34. Council of Teaching Hospitals, Association of American Medical Colleges, *Toward a More Contemporary Public Understanding of the Teaching Hospital*. Washington, D.C.: May 1979, p. 10.
35. Sheps, Clark *et al.*, *op. cit.*, p. 12.
36. Council of Teaching Hospitals, *op. cit.*, p. 3. Association of American Medical Colleges, *op. cit.*, p. 16, Fig. 14.
37. Council of Teaching Hospitals, *op. cit.*, p. 3. *Hospital Statistics*, 1980 Edition. Chicago: American Hospitals Assoc., p. 178, Table 8.
38. *Hospital Statistics*, 1980 Edition, *op. cit.*, p. 184, Table 10A; p. 178, Table 8.
39. Council of Teaching Hospitals, *op. cit.*, pp. 39 ff.
40. Personal Communication. Blue Cross/Blue Shield of North Carolina, 1980.
41. Council of Teaching Hospitals, *op. cit.*, p. 45.
42. D. E. Rogers, *American Medicine: Challenge for the 1980s*. Cambridge: Ballinger, 1978, p. 66.
43. Association of American Medical Colleges, *op. cit.*, p. 12, Fig. 3.
44. A. W. Snoke, "The Teaching Hospital—Its Responsibilities and Conflicts," *Journal of Medical Education*, Vol. 35 (March 1960), pp. 207-213.
45. Sheps, Clark, *et al.*, *op. cit.*, pp. 29 ff.
46. Council of Teaching Hospitals, *op. cit.*, p. 10.
47. G. P. Berry in S. J. Axelrod, F. Goldmann, J. N. Muller, C. G. Sheps, and M. Terris (eds.), *Readings in Medical Care*. Chapel Hill: University of North Carolina Press, 1958, p. VI.
48. D. E. Rogers and R. J. Blendon, "The Academic Medical Center: A Stressed Institution," *New England Journal of Medicine*, Vol. 298, No. 17. (April 27, 1978), pp. 940-950.
49. J. A. D. Cooper, "Medical Centers: Looking to the Future," *Journal of Medical Education*, Vol. 50 (Jan. 1975), pp. 92-94.

Chapter 3

The Delivery of Health Services and the Academic Medical Center

IMPORTANCE OF PATIENT CARE IN ACADEMIC MEDICAL CENTERS

The role of the academic medical centers in the delivery of health services to individual communities and the nation at large requires further delineation. Almost 1,000 of the nation's hospitals have some type of affiliation involving programmed education activities. The 792 community hospitals with such affiliations tend to be the larger hospitals. They account for 40 percent of the total hospital beds and provide care for 30 percent of community hospital out patient and emergency visits.

While the centers continue faithfully to recite the familiar litany of their traditional threefold mission of education, research, and patient care, there is great tension, uncertainty, and conflict within the university about the proper balance and the priorities to be accorded to each goal and, in truth, about what the missions and goals ought to be. In fact, it is increasingly clear that the function of patient care as traditionally viewed by the medical faculty is not synonymous with delivery of health services. These considerations are well recognized in the academic centers. A 1980 report on the organization and governance

79

of academic health centers, conducted by the Association of Academic Health Centers (AAHC), noted that:

> Most faculty members currently in academic health centers entered when the model resembled a research university and the emphasis was on teaching and research. Patient care was considered part of the teaching program, and faculty usually were not appointed solely on the basis of teaching expertise. Service responsibilities, especially in delivering ambulatory and primary patient care, have increased dramatically in the last ten years. Patient care and community services are now dominant forces in shaping the mission of most academic health centers.[1]

The emphasis on service has grown without strategic or community health planning, reflecting needs that are inherent in the programs and interests of the centers rather than the needs of a population per se. Centers see the increases in patient care activity either as a necessary (though perhaps grudging) response to demands from surrounding populations or as a means toward teaching and training goals. In any case, the delivery of health services represents an important source of revenue to maintain faculty and support other programs.

Surely Abraham Flexner had no large patient care and health service complexes in mind when his 1910 report urged that medical schools control selected hospitals in order to improve bedside teaching of medical students. Whatever the theoretically ideal balance of medical center functions, there is little doubt that the provision of services to large aggregations of patients and the concurrent training of specialists which such services makes possible are major driving forces in today's academic medical center.

FROM PATIENT CARE TO DELIVERY OF HEALTH SERVICES

Full comprehension of this development at academic medical centers requires an appreciation of several factors that influence access to medical care and the delivery of health services.[2] First, medical care is so different from other elements of our social and economic system that society has found it cannot rely upon the medical marketplace alone for its receipt and delivery. Instead, we rely heavily on public policy to assure the interventions required to fulfill the needs of the population. Thus, as we have set forth in Chapter 1, government has supported both the development of human and physical resources and the advancement of biomedical science, and has steadily moved to eliminate financial and organizational barriers to the delivery of health services.

Second, the range of personal problems brought to physicians reflects the marked tensions and stresses that individuals encounter in this dynamic, pressure-laden society. The problems that the physician is called upon to solve involve much more than organic disease. He or she often needs the help of other professionals, nonmedical as well as medical. At the same time, the physician has to avoid the easy assumption that ready answers to these problems are to be found in the technical weapons that science, with the help of society, has made so abundantly available.

Finally, as discussed in Chapter 1, the strategies of public policy for improving access to health services at reasonable cost are unlikely to succeed if they are developed as solutions to isolated or independent issues. Corrections to one part of the health system cannot be made effectively unless the implications for other parts are taken into account.

Delivery of health services is probably the most complex and controversial arena of health policy. In comparison with the fields of research and medical education, there are fewer generally recognized, widely accepted norms. Health services policy compels examination of deeply held values and deals with gigantic financial stakes. Moreover, to the old propaganda issue of "socialized medicine" has now been added political cynicism and mistrust of government and planning. It will be no simple task to harmonize faculty aspirations for the academic medical center with the developments in public policy for health services.

Medical care aims to prevent and cure illness, treat pain, and restore the afflicted to optimum functioning capacity. No longer can man always find the relief he seeks from informal and simple sources of help. Instead, he must more often turn to the formal sources of large-scale organizations, including the academic medical center. This inevitably means involvement with the modern bureaucracy, which may be impersonal and even inaccessible to the needs of people under stress. Medicine thus finds itself an essential part of a broad social support system for society. Beyond the function of *curing* by applying the technology so characteristic of modern medicine is the *caring* function relevant at all times, but particularly crucial in primary care.

All too often medical care is defined in terms only of the practice of clinical medicine, i.e., the task of the individual physician to diagnose, treat, and cure. Essentially, this is the framework used for medical education in the academic medical center. And therein lies the heart of the paradox that service delivery has become such a driving force of the academic center. For medical care (or "health service") is actually a complex consisting of three large components. The first is the individuals and families who demand or need personal health services. These demands and needs will vary by age, culture, geography, income, sex, and previous health status. The second component is the health care profession: doctors, nurses, pharmacists, and millions of other trained health workers.

But the major elements of the health system are highly organized, institutionalized, and centralized as a third component, which makes possible the interaction between patient and professional. This is a social component, which we call the organization, delivery, and financing of medical care. How we organize health services, where these services are delivered, how we then pay for them, and what technology we buy are distinct but interrelated questions. The answers are found in the large-scale organizations and institutions that define our public/private pluralistic health care system. The task of this social component is to arrange the interaction betwen the patient and the health system so as to (1) minimize the barriers to access by the patient; (2) maximize the quality of care that he receives; and (3) assure a reasonable cost to the patient and society. This task and the interaction among the three components are represented schematically in Figure 1.[3]

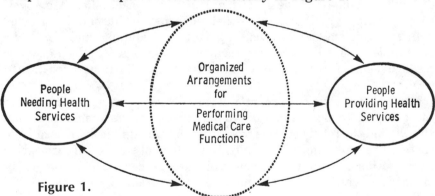

Figure 1.

This social component has increasingly become the focus of public policy during the past thirty to forty years. It cannot be made rational by the marketplace alone. The conviction has developed, especially in government and among third-party payers, that major improvements in health care delivery can and should be made. At bottom, we find that none of the major issues—resource allocation, technology assessment, manpower distribution, or changing attitudes towards health services—can be dealt with effectively except in terms of determining the scope of and responsibility for organizing health services. This requires not only ensuring financial coverage of defined populations but also clarifying the levels of primary, secondary, and tertiary care and regionalizing facilities where appropriate. Financial entitlement to care and availability of appropriate sources of care should go hand in hand.

The academic medical center finds itself in the center of this swirling controversy over the delivery of health services. It surely never bargained for this, although the educational reforms stimulated by the Flexner report moved it slowly in this direction. In large measure, this new position of the academic medical center reflects the impact of external influences upon academic medicine. Substantial governmental funds for both clinical training and research and development along categorical disease lines surely speeded the development of medical specialization. This largesse, especially from the National Institutes of Health, each interested in specific disease categories, helped to transfer primary faculty interest from the education of undergraduate students to the training of residents in graduate medical education, to the further training of specialists and subspecialists, and to the development of research and the technological armament to fight disease. These new faculty interests could only be furthered by the aggregation of patients with the relevant diseases in appropriate volume.

In recent years a broader, more persistent, and less differentiated external influence has been the health status of the population of the neighboring community. Although the precise geographical extent of the relevant community is seldom well defined, it nevertheless represents a force that the center cannot ignore, precisely because it is the obvious major, often the largest, human resource for health care services. Unlike the governmental influences for education, training, and research, community pressure is uniquely concerned with the broad spectrum of health services. This pressure has growing support from state and local governments.

The academic medical center is acutely aware of these factors and of the impact of external influences on its mission and goals. In its report on organization and governance, for example, the Association of Academic Health Centers noted some significant changes:

4. Since the 1960's the academic health centers have been required to assume a larger role in providing basic health care services in their own communities. On the one hand, expanding technology and research funds have contributed to the development of advanced medical capabilities, have produced numerous sub-specialties, and have turned academic health centers into the principal source of tertiary care. On the other hand, there has been a major thrust in this country to provide more and better care to the elderly, and, in recent years, considerable social political pressure on academic health centers to provide some

primary care to consumers in the areas they serve.

5. Academic health centers also have been affected by a significant
increase in the regulation of their practices and procedures by all
levels of government. As health care became a major political-social
issue, academic health centers evolved from rather autonomous institutions into a key element in a highly regulated and very controversial industry...[4]

External influences will intensify in future years but they will not
be welcomed by academic medicine. An AAHC survey of the attitudes
of the principal officials in the academic health centers clearly reveal-
ed academic medicine's apprehensions about government intervention.
Although increased demands for primary and secondary care are
definitely anticipated, the greatest concern of the centers is their growing uncertainty about how effectively the traditional teaching hospital
will render tertiary care. Especially unwelcome will be politically imposed requirements that may increasingly accompany payment for services to patients, e.g., restrictions on the size of payments, coverage
of the costs for graduate medical education, or fee payments for the
services of full-time faculty physicians.

In essence, the function of "patient care" has been overtaken and
paralleled by the concept of the "delivery of health services," which
has always made academic medicine uncomfortable. In contrast with
the clinician's application of skill and knowledge to diagnose and cure
an individual patient's disease, the delivery of health services embraces
the full range of health needs of aggregate populations and of
geographical communities. Academic medicine has never been much
interested in the health needs of communities or pupulations per se.
This has been left to the fields of public health and the social and
behavorial sciences. But as academic disciplines, these fields have no
power to minister directly to these changing needs. It is only when they
are organized as operating units in hospitals or departments of government (e.g., health departments) that they can do more than explain the
needs or bring attention to them.

RELATIONSHIP OF HEALTH SERVICES
TO EDUCATION AND TRAINING

Clearly, changes in health needs and demographic alterations over
the past several decades call for vast modifications in the practice of
medicine. They demand the management of the chronically or mentally ill and more attention to the aged, wherein medicine cannot stand

alone. They call for the organization and provision of primary care, which particularly requires a functional interdisciplinary format. The academic medical center cannot be responsible for health services delivery to all, but it is responsible for setting the pattern to meet these needs. This it has not yet overtly done. In their concentration on second-dary and tertiary care, medical education and research focus on the process and etiology of disease, principally from the biological point of view. The teaching hospital continues to emphasize the care of the acutely ill patient, especially during the inpatient phase.

Prevailing medical school philosophy would limit the responsibility of the clinical faculty for patient care to the level needed to support the dominant research and education functions and interests. Faculty discussions about an appropriate balance of functions contain vague references, comforting to the faculty, to "quality" and "excellence," but these discussions are substantially irrelevant to the reality of the pressures for service. Academic debate rarely asks "Whom does this quality serve?" "Education for what?" "How does medical education as we provide it specifically affect the future practice of medicine?"[5]

The academic medical center has become a multimillion dollar enterprise fundamentally dependent for its fiscal and its programmatic survival upon a constant stream of acutely ill patients—an aggregation representing as much as possible the research and teaching interests of many groups of faculty members. Without this aggregation, the modern careers of academic clinicians in research and training would be impossible—or so it seems to them. The traditional emphasis on inpatient services persists, while outpatient departments and emergency rooms, despite some improvements in the past fifteen years, remain the Siberia of the hospital and are considered a second-class teaching environment.

These realities of the modern academic medical center have important implications for health services and health costs which the centers must eventually deal with realistically and constructively. At the same time, there are equally serious implications for medical education, as we shall discuss in Chapter 4. The examination of these implications and the development of new approaches to both the delivery of services and medical education must go forward simultaneously. For the attitudes and aspirations of the medical profession are stimulated and fashioned in the education process. As one of the authors said nearly ten years ago,

> Education and training and the delivery of service are inextricably inter-
> woven... From its educational responsibilities, the medical school thus
> derives its responsibility to help organize the service system and to deliver

care in that system. Education in primary care requires its own environment.[6]

The predicament of the academic medical center has recently won greater recognition, but some medical educators were well aware of it long ago. Although medical schools tried to ignore continued and rapid changes in social forces during their own development into large-scale academic medical centers, some academic leaders at the 1965 Institute on the Medical Center and the University, sponsored by the Association of American Medical Colleges, foreshadowed today's problems. Ward Darley, who was formerly dean of the College of Medicine and president of the University of Colorado, cited a number of "future inevitables," and Robert Ebert, then dean of the Harvard Medical School, expressed his doubts that the medical schools were adequately organized to deal with the service function.

Obviously, there is no simple formula for adjusting the traditional emphasis on education, research, and patient care in specialty medicine so as to meet the current deficiencies in primary care services for individuals, families, and communities. The medical center is justifiably concerned with the financial risks inherent in a strictly service operation given the inadequacies of today's third-party coverage as to eligibility for benefits, level of payment, or service rendered. As the AAHC report put it, "the problem of health services, which and how much, will undoubtedly increase tension within the health center but especially with the rest of the university community."[7]

ACCESS, PAYMENTS, AND COSTS

Public policy actions are needed to help academic medical centers solve their dilemma. But these will not be easy to formulate. First, there is a popular view that technology in medicine may have arrived at a point of diminishing returns, a view that is accompanied by a kind of "medical populism" in which "consumerism" plays a prominent role. Second, there is a mood approaching a policy consensus that health care costs ought to be contained. These two attitudes explain much of the increasing divergence between the medical faculties' concept of the centers' service role and the view held by their political (i.e., budgetary) supporters. This gulf in perception has to be bridged.

Again, as we have seen, the history of health policy has been one of attempting to expand access to health care, presumptively to make the benefits of modern scientific medicine readily available to everyone. Both public and private studies show clear progress. The trend in the past decade has been toward more equitable access, more equal use of physician and hospital services, wider coverage of the costs of health care, and improvements in the health status of populations.[8] The poor and the elderly especially have made substantial gains via the Medicare and Medicaid programs in both their financial access to the their use of health services. Improvements in life expectancy and declines in infant mortality have been especially noticeable since 1965.

Nevertheless, serious gaps remain. It has been officially estimated that 12.6 percent of the civilian noninstitutionalized population, or 26.6 million people, have no third-party coverage whatever.[9] As Louise Russell noted in a recent report of The Brookings Institution, "Despite the new programs and the large expenditures, not everyone is covered, not everyone shares in the abundance, and many people can still draw up long lists of needs that remain to be filled."[10] President Carter's 1980 National Health Plan had estimated that, apart from those persons without any insurance coverage, an additional 19 million to 46 million have insurance that is inadequate either as to ordinary medical services or as to catastrophic illness costs. Some 51 million persons were estimated to reside in "medically underserved" urban and rural areas with few or no physicians or other resources for primary care services. In the past, federal and state public policy has supported the creation and organization of a range of community health services to meet this gap—neighborhood and family health centers, maternity and infant care centers, family planning services, community mental health centers, and mental retardation centers. The National Health Service Corps is the most recent national effort of this sort. It differs from the others in assigning health personnel directly to needy areas on a voluntary basis or as means of paying back medical school scholarships.

But by 1980 both the past accomplishments of the health care system and the efforts needed to fill the remaining gaps were overshadowed by concern about the nation's general economic condition and the continually increasing proportion of national resources spent on health care, rather than of any precise evaluation of public attitudes. Surveys generally show that patients are not highly critical of their own medical care. One survey reflected an overall rate of patient satisfaction of 88 percent. Not unexpectedly, the area of greatest dissatisfaction seems to be cost; on this issue, the rate of satisfaction fell to 63 percent. At the same time, 61 percent of the respondents paradoxically seem to believe that the medical care system is in crisis, the nature of which is not clearly expressed.[11] Whatever the factual base, it seems undeniable that the cornerstone for evaluating future courses of action by government will be the issue of health care costs, both total health care costs and total public spending for health and other purposes.

As policymakers look to the academic medical centers to fill service gaps in a framework of cost constraints, they are confronted with several paradoxes. The centers are clearly the linchpins of the hospital system in each state and in major urban areas. But through their outpatient departments and emergency rooms they have unwillingly become the family doctor for millions of poor urban Americans of all races and ages. Although urban minority populations, for example, report that they increasingly have found a regular source of medical care, they are more than five times as likely as nonminorities to find that source in a hospital outpatient department or emergency room, usually a public general hospital affiliated with a medical school.[12] In addition, the academic medical centers, heavily concentrated in metropolitan areas like New York, Philadelphia, Chicago, and Dallas, have experienced a substantial loss of certain types of patients to the suburbs, where graduates of academic medical center residency training programs provide specialist care of top quality. This loss of paying or insured patients has had a serious impact not only on the workload of the full-time clinical faculty but also on their capacity to maintain their specialist training programs. Finally, the centers have experienced fiscal constraints expecially in states like New York where cost control programs are extensive.

At the same time, academic medical centers resist interdigitation with the community and the regionalization or rationalization of high-cost, sophisticated, technologically oriented specialist services. Each center continues to fight for its own individual jurisdiction for all health services rather than for interinstitutional agreements to share high-cost services. This pattern is particularly marked at the most prestigious institutions, which by definition are the most costly.

In brief, the academic medical center resembles other aggregate noncorporate institutions in its resistance to change and insistence on self-preservation and survival in its present form. The heart of the problem is that the patient care and specialist training programs of each academic medical center have developed in response to internal demands and independent of planning for the health needs of the public. True, many centers have come to deal with community needs, but usually only under duress. Thus their actions were often taken piecemeal and without enthusiasm. Occasionally an academic medical center will sponsor a health maintenance organization or a neighborhood health center, but this is usually a separate organization. Health services at the academic medical center have been regarded by academic medicine as its own preserve, not necessarily to be fitted into the framework of the general health care system.

Against this background of emerging policy to control costs while filling service gaps, academic medical centers approach this set of paradoxes almost wholly from a fiscal standpoint. Almost all academic medical centers are preoccupied with generating large amounts of revenue from faculty private clinical practice as a way to make up for constraints on government research and education grants and contracts. The service functions of the academic medical centers and the efforts now under way to use and expand them as a major revenue source thus raise several significant questions about the interaction between the centers and public policy. These principal issues are:

1. How will the new or expanded clinical services bear upon the policies of controlling costs?
2. What precise role should be played by the health services programs of the academic medical center as the United States moves towards a rationally organized health care system?
3. What are the strengths, weaknesses, tensions, and pressures within the academic medical centers as they attempt to deal with these questions of health services delivery?

Can we move to a more rational health care system in the United States and develop a long-term cost containment strategy without the clear and overt involvement of the academic medical center? Are changes called for in the way academic medical centers are organized, governed, and managed? The answers to these questions will come only partly from academe, and partly from the domain of public policy.

GROWING FACULTY PRACTICE

Medical school faculty members traditionally treated private patients in medical school facilities and teaching hospitals under informal arrangements that provided varying personal income supplements. After World War II, however, when clinical faculty steadily shifted to the status of salaried, full-time faculty, and public and private insurance made large and lucrative clinical practices possible, medical center leadership moved to replace the informal arrangements with mechanisms known as faculty practice plans.

The terms and conditions of these plans, the options or requirements, as the case might be, for faculty clinical practice, and the division of clinical earnings among faculty, departments, and center administration have been the source of numerous problems and much intrauniversity conflict. Many deans have been unseated in the process of confrontation over the distribution of clinical earnings and the extent to which such earnings could or should support the overall budget of the academic medical center.

The last in a series of AAMC reports on faculty practice plans issued in 1977 stated:

> This review has reinforced the contention that no subject concerning medical school management has led to more agony and heated debate among the schools' administrators and faculty than that concerning the form and operation of service plans. The issue—thorny to say the least at many schools—has contributed to the departure of deans and presidents, has brought about serious impasses between clinical faculty and medical school managers, and has triggered great concern over which institutional mission should predominate—education or service.[13]

While the installation of large-scale faculty practice plans is not a new development in academic medical centers, their expansion today and the apparent intention that such plans become a major source of medical school financing raise concerns as to how the public interest is served. Income derived from faculty practice has risen from about 3 percent of the total income of the nation's medical schools to about 15 percent. This income relates only to medical school budgets. Hospitals and other patient care facilities of the centers also contributed substantial, if unreported, amounts to the support of faculty and other medical school costs. Radiology, anesthesiology, and pathology, the traditional hospital-based specialties, are only a case in point. Many hospitals cover the salaries of full-time clinical faculty in surgery, medicine, and pediatrics, the cost of which must be met from clinical practice, not research or training grants. In any case, the reported figures undoubtedly represent only a part of the actual income of medical school faculty practice, which could range as high as $1.8 billion.[14]

The special interests of the academic medical center have led it to move aggressively to find new sources of funds to offset government budget cuts threatening their rate of growth, the maintenance of faculty and other personnel, and the replacement of old equipment. Unfortunately, the inevitable consequences of expanding the clinical practice of faculty will be medical price inflation and an increase in total medical care costs. Levels of payment by insurers (excluding Medicaid) under the prevailing fee-for-service method of payment are most commonly determined by a system of "usual, customary, and reasonable" charges. Under UCR, a physician's *future* fee profile is established on the basis of his *past* charges and those of other physicians in the same specialty. The incentive is then both strong and unavoidable for physicians to bill consistently at higher rates. In addition, the UCR reflects the usual pattern of higher fees for procedurally oriented subspecialist medical care.[15] Since such care is the hallmark of every academic medical center, expansion of faculty practice, particularly where it involves elective procedures, can lead only to total higher costs.

Thus it would seem that the medical centers are ignoring, at their peril, the implications for public policy in the area of cost control and containment. They also ignore the unfavorable public reaction to disclosures of very high physician income. The American public is fully aware of and concerned about the continued growth of national health expenditures.

By now we have surely come to regard as rather old-fashioned the idea, as Reinhardt put it, that physician and patient can between them decide "what treatment is to be applied and someone pays for it (presumably at the physician's usual and customary rate of hourly income)."[16] Rather, by "socializing" the payment for health services, whether through public or private insurance mechanisms, we have come to a broad social consensus relative to continued growth of health expenses. Again, as Louise Russell has said, "Trying to do everything worthwhile means escalating costs. Controlling costs means going without."[17] All Western nations have had to learn this same lesson, namely, the problem of choice—among services, among regions, among populations. As in all social endeavors, "the final common denominator is money, its expenditure and its return."[18]

In the future, the main issue for the academic medical center, as for all other elements of the health system, will be the control of money. The role of the public sector is central because it pays so much of the bill, and all indications are that cost control measures applicable to all sources of payment, public and private, insurance and fee-for-service, will become more, not less, stringent. It would be naive for academic medical centers to believe that extensive ventures intended to enlarge faculty clinical practice income can long elude public policy on cost control.

CONTAINMENT OF HEALTH CARE COSTS

Concern about health costs now overshadows all elements of the debate over national health insurance. The advocacy so widely expressed in the 1960s and early 1970s of breaking down financial and organizational barriers to health care has been paralleled, if not already replaced, by assertions that the nation cannot "afford" national health insurance. This issue of affordability embraces not only the scope and timing of expansion of benefit coverage but also the sources of financing, i.e., public versus private. Regrettably, there seems to be little recognition that the effectiveness of the mechanisms of control and administration will largely determine whether national health insurance is in fact affordable.[19]

National health insurance can take many forms, the details of which need not detain us here. It is ironic that academic medicine, despite its programmatic dependence on health services and its fiscal dependence on the outcome of public policy on cost control, should have contributed so little to the debate over national health insurance, in terms of either relevant research or participation in the policy debates. Whether the plans have limited benefit coverage (e.g., catastrophic medical costs) or extensive coverage (e.g., full ambulatory and inpatient care), a limited or an extensive federal role, a voluntary or mandated private insurance role, the consensus has been reached that cost is a fundamental political constraint on any approach to national health insurance. In light of their dominant position in health care, it is surely strange that academic medical centers tend to stand aside from the debate, arguing only that their unique functions and accompanying high-cost teaching hospitals should be fully supported in their present form. The centers are fully aware that they have a significant impact on gross health expenditures. Their hospital affiliations are extensive, their teaching hospitals are high cost, their focus is on new technology, their outpatient departments provide ambulatory care at high cost, and now they are expanding their practice plans.

The precise form of cost control policies to which medical center service plans must accommodate is, of course, not yet set. For some ten years the nation, the states, and the insurance plans or carriers have acted without a comprehensive policy of cost containment. Although there has been a great deal of activity and some experimentation, most efforts have been attempts to deal piecemeal with single payers or types of payers or providers or patients. These efforts have fallen into three main categories. One has been the control of utilization through various kinds of monitoring and the promotion of new methods of organizing and delivering health care services, such as requiring second surgical opinions, increasing insurance deductibles, and sponsoring health maintenance organizations. A second area is health resources planning and development, with special stress, of late, on technology assessment, creation of some 200 health system agencies (HSAs) to cover the nation, and the control or certification of need for capital investment by HSAs and other local and state health planning agencies. Finally, we have moved to develop specific reimbursement controls, in some states creating agencies that set hospital rates and physician fees, and supporting Medicare/Medicaid reimbursement experiments. Although there is some effort at voluntary hospital cost control, attempts to institute a mandatory national hospital cost control law have failed.[20]

Cost containment efforts thus far have not been greatly effective. Many thoughtful students of the problem believe that the most successful programs will be those that set a limit on total resources through budgeting or similar prospective restraints. We have learned that cost control policies must obviously be related to our goals in the delivery of care, e.g., access for all, including quality of care, and goals in education and research. We face a seamless web of considerations in determining the allocation of resources for health. We have come to understand that, in the final analysis, cost issues are issues of budget, and as in all budgetary matters, the decision makers must judge the return or the benefit resulting from proposed health expenditures.

But in the health field such judgements are not made simply or easily. The outcome or results of health expenditures are not always quantifiable. Moreover, policymakers, like the average citizen, are increasingly skeptical of the adequacy and performance of the health care system, including the value of high expenditures for the new technologies.

Cost issues are often actually financing issues. Revenue is the opposite side of the coin of costs. Thus, when a physician's fees are controlled or fixed by law or third-party payers, but he remains free to accept the fee as full payment or not, he is likely to shift his patient load or the charge to the source of revenue that will pay his fee, usually the patient himself. Thus cost as such remains unaffected. If we expect the teaching hospital to care for the poor, then the poor must have appropriate insurance or other coverage to pay the hospital for its services. When Medicaid rates are arbitarily set regardless of the cost of meeting service needs, hospital deficits occur. Costs per se are not necessarily controlled; they are merely shifted to other payers.

All health care providers and all payers of the costs of care are concerned about continued cost escalation, but each interest tries to protect its own financial position by various disconnected measures that may or may not restrict the total costs. For example, hospitals and physicians are mainly concerned with *revenue* and thus try to establish a high *price*—or charge or fee—and enlarge the volume of utilization. In contrast, third-party insurance payers are mainly concerned with reasonable *costs*, especially of hospitals, because they account for the largest single item of health expenditures. But like hospitals and physicians, they focus only upon their own share of the cost. Consequently, Medicare excludes many hospital costs in its rules on allowable costs because they are not incurred for the elderly. The effect is to reduce Medicare expenses but the hospital must turn to other sources if the disallowed costs are essential. Because of the interplay of these forces, the impact of present cost control policies is largely to shift the burden of costs among payers, eventually to the individual patient himself. Indeed, this idea of "cost-sharing" by the patient is the thrust of much of the argument for competition in health care financing and delivery.

Effective cost containment will obviously mean that we cannot have all that is regarded as useful or worthwhile. We may have to reduce hospital beds, limit freedom to practice by specialty or to choose a physician, provide "paybacks" for National Health Service Corps service in medically underserved areas, and phase in or control the rate of technological applications. In this context, the intentions of academic medicine to expand medical practice plans face serious questioning.

LIMITATIONS OF FACULTY PRACTICE

An increase in the volume of clinical practice at academic medical centers, if it is inspired primarily as a financing device, will probably hurt primary care services, which yield lower fees. Current efforts at primary care education, research, and care will be seriously eroded. This eventuality was forecast in the 1974 Rand Corporation study of the impact of federal manpower legislation medical schools. The Rand report concluded:

> If medical school deans seek to compensate for federal cutbacks by increasing institutional revenue from faculty practice, as we expect they will, the education and care programs of the clinical departments will be directly affected. The structure of third-party reimbursement for professional services is such that the surgical and procedurally oriented medical subspecialties have the greatest earning capacity particularly in the academic health centers. To increase revenue from patient care, the composition of the patient population in the teaching hospitals will have to shift to include more patients who require the services of the high paying specialists. The shift will necessitate more concentration on secondary and tertiary care and less on primary care. Other things equal, faculty growth in the clinical departments can also be expected to favor the high earning specialties, those generally not involved in primary care. [21]

At the same time, it cannot be assumed that the academic medical center will abandon primary care. On the contrary, even if its motivations are financial, the center will presumably have to provide enough primary care to feed the specialty services. Such primary care, however, will clearly be carried out in the most expensive way if only because the centers are neither equipped nor motivated to provide quality primary care efficiently.

As government tries to make the service functions of the academic medical center more consonant with the public interest, it will be accused of regulating medical education. But the object of the regulation is what goes on in the teaching hospital and its service environment: excessive specialization, high costs, excessive and unevaluated technology, and inadequate attention to the community, especially where the teaching hospital is its major medical resource. The effort to generate practice income thus exposes the current inner trends and tensions within the academic medical center between the medical school and the hospital, whose patient care activities have been modified by academic needs for teaching and research but whose primary mission will increasingly be seen as service.

As Robert Ebert, president of the Milbank Memorial Fund and former dean of the Harvard Medical School, has argued, in their zeal to be academic, many teaching hospitals have stressed their functions as a referral center, especially for tertiary care. They have exercised little leadership in introducing new technologies into practice on a broad scale and testing their effectiveness, economy, and quality. They have had scant interest in innovations for providing personal health services, especially in primary care.[22] To be a referral center for tertiary care on as broad a front as possible, regardless of other available resources, remains the driving ambition of almost all academic centers.

The service function, especially the new emphasis on faculty practice income, thus raises a number of internal management and policy issues for the medical center. As total health costs rise, financing agencies are likely to insist upon an effective separation of cost and funding for research, education, and patient care. Such separation will put great pressure on tuition levels for undergraduate medical education as well as sources of funding for residency training. Cost increases at hospitals in academic medical centers above expected cost containment norms could lead to tight reimbursement controls over the training of specialists and restrictions on the introduction of new technologies. Inevitably, there will be internal school and university conflict over control of various types of funds, especially that generated by clinical faculty, whose power is bound to increase vis-a-vis other faculty and the administration, as the amounts generated by clinical practice increase.

Within the clinical faculty there could well be a strong movement away from teaching fulltime. We can envision a further weakening of the position of the dean and the basic science faculty; at the same time, the management of the teaching hospital and satellite service programs or practice plans will become more powerful as well as more professional.

As these tensions surface, there will be protracted debates about the nature and clarity of mission and purpose in the medical center. Above all, the centers will have to deal with issues relating to the scope, organization, efficiency, and effectiveness of the services they provide. The traditional trinity of functions—education, research and patient care—will need reexamination as the medical school and funding agencies ask, in Sheps's terms, "Education for What?"[23] Moreover, health care management and finance, government relations, epidemiological expressions of health care priorities—these will, in time, need to become dominant factors in academic medicine. There will have to be changes in the training of physicians if they are to practice effectively in an environment where such issues are important. The academic medical center will not be able to relegate them fully to offices of administration or departments of community health.

Generally, if present trends in faculty practice continue, we can expect raging academic controversy over the status and rank of those faculty members who increase their clinical functions at the expense of traditional academic activity. The tension between the scholars and the physicians spending more time in patient care will mount, as will the disparity between the two parties in income. We can anticipate much unhappiness among basic biomedical scientists, especially if they become dependent, even to a degree, upon the earnings of clinical faculty for the support of their research.

DEREGULATION AND COMPETITION

The current approach of the academic medical center to the delivery of health services is essentially entrepreneurial and fiscal. The concern of academic medicine for the substance of medical diagnosis, treatment, and cure has now been matched by its increasing expertise in the intricacies of reimbursement for services. To a fair degree, current attitudes are the logical outcome of the public policy initiated with the enactment of Medicare and Medicaid in 1965, under which academic medical centers are reimbursed for hospital and physician services they had traditionally provided without charge to those unable to pay. This entrepreneurial approach is also consistent with the current swing in public attitudes and the enactment of new legislation favoring competition in the society at large. Principles of deregulation of industry in favor of competition have already been enacted in regard to aviation, truck transport, and railroads, and undoubtedly will be enacted in other fields of industrial activity as well as human services programs.

The alleged virtues of competition are now often advanced in the field of health and medicine. The choice seems to be developing between, on the one hand, techniques of government regulation and legislative mandates to structure and organize a national health system and, on the other, reliance on competition, supported by government stimuli, legislative and financial. It is not clear yet which choice will be adopted, but competition and marketplace economics are getting increasing Congressional attention. In February 1980 the Subcommittee on Health of the U.S. House Ways and Means Committee held public hearings on various legislative proposals to restructure incentives in the private health sector that might encourage cost control by stimulating competition and greater cost consciousness among patients and providers. These proposals generally take the approach of requiring increased consumer cost-sharing through deductibles and coinsurance and of tying eligibility of insurance plans for tax benefits to provisions for co-insurance and sizable out-of-pocket expenditures.[24] The most extensive proposal in the past few years to restore or enhance competition and still achieve national health objectives was the Consumer-Choice Health Plan advanced by Alain Enthoven during the Carter Administration.[25] As of this writing, the Reagan administration has not made specific proposals for Congressional action.

The 1979 Congressional amendments to P.L. 93-641, the National Health Planning and Resources Development Act, include three clear endorsements of the principle of competition in the health planning process. These endorsements added:

1. A new national planning priority of strengthening competition where it would help in quality assurance, cost effectiveness, and access to care.
2. A new purpose for local Health Systems Agencies to preserve or improve competition.
3. Two additional review criteria stressing competition in the HSA review of plans and projects.[26]

This heightened Congressional concern with competition is not unnoticed at the academic medical center. In its *Weekly Reports,* the Association of American Medical Colleges officially advises teaching hospitals to think about how they will fare in a price-competitive environment. As academic centers take stock of these new developements, they are being told in the *Journal of Medical Education* of the Association of American Medical Colleges to develop "marketing strategies." Such strategies, says the author, will enable teaching hospitals to compete effectively with community hospitals to which they are now losing patient referrals because they no longer have a monopoly on high-quality specialty patient care formerly available only at major teaching hospitals.[27]

At the same time, centers will find that no matter what mix of competition and regulation emerges as public policy, it will be aimed at decreasing the flow of funds into the health care system. Even if government enacts measures to enhance competition among private insurers and still assures adequate coverage for the poor or for the costs of catastrophic illness, academic medical centers will face very serious problems in adjusting to a so-called "price competitive environment." In the first place, the centers may well discover that they cannot survive competitively without substantial curtailment of the expensive tertiary-care services on which they now focus. Alternatively, if the total resources become very limited, the *volume* of needed care may diminish very substantially. Surely, if price is to become a controlling criterion in the selection of a hospital, many supporting and back-up social services will have to be abandoned by academic medical centers, thus affecting the quality of care. On the other hand, if teaching hospitals confined their services entirely to tertiary care, they would be an even more artificial and unrealistic environment for medical education than they are now. And if academic medical centers had to rely on competitive medical practice plans and the health maintenance organization (HMO) form of health care delivery, with its stress on cost controls, they would probably find it impossible to finance training in primary care.[28]

PRIMARY CARE: POLICIES AND PARADOXES

To date, there has been little indication that any new emphasis on competition as the keynote of future public policy will be accompanied by a recognition of the unique importance of the academic medical center to the health system as a whole. Certainly, there has been no evident interest in how new policies and practices may affect the center's role in preparing physicians to practice primary care. Our own observation is that government has not yet grasped the uniqueness of the academic medical center. Instead, the tendency is to regard the centers as no more than another special interest pressing upon government for their own welfare. Senior officials in the National Institutes of Health, the Health Care Financing Administration, Health Resources Administration, and other parts of the Public Health Service in the Department of Health and Human Services never meet collectively to review the impact on academic medical centers of their separate but related policies. Thus far, they view the current enlargement of medical center private practice plans as entirely a fiscal venture aimed at survival alone. The implications of this development for delivery of health services, especially primary care, are totally ignored.

We find this policy of inattention both paradoxical and dangerous. It must be viewed against a history of public policy developments that have pressed very hard for more extensive primary care services within an expanding health care system. The insistent demand for such services has been fueled by the enactment of Medicare and Medicaid, the changing nature of the burden of disease, and rapid population shifts between regions of the country and urban or rural areas. More than 1700 primary care health manpower shortage areas have been identified by the Department of Health and Human Services. Over 37 million people, 15 percent of the nation's population, reside in these areas.[29]

To meet these needs, Congress and the states have, over the past fifteen years, supported a number of innovative programs in service delivery, e.g., neighborhood and other primary health centers, the Rural Health Initative, and the National Health Service Corps. Additionally, they have attempted to deal with the facts of geographic and specialty distribution by offering incentives as well as mandates for the primary care education and manpower training programs of the academic medical center. Beyond tying student assistance funds to potential service in shortage areas, policymakers have provided for area health education centers under the aegis of the academic medical center, expanded opportunities for the growth of the specialty of family medicine, and increased residency positions in the primary care fields of family practice, internal medicine, and pediatrics.

In their own turn, policymakers should be aware that primary care represents much more than a challenge to the academic medical center to meet societal needs. Rather, the emphasis on primary care constitutes perhaps the most ominous threat to the hallowed traditions of the academic medical center—at least those traditions encouraged in the last half century of biomedical scientific progress. There has developed a widespread consensus that a more balanced health care system requires a higher proportion and better distribution of primary care physicians.[30]

The terms used to describe the levels of personal health care—primary, secondary, and tertiary—are admittedly imprecise and overlapping. Indeed, solid, unchanging, and impermeable lines of differentiation are not desirable. Nevertheless, each level has a distinguishable focus and scope of responsibility. Primary care should provide the essential and continuing contact between the individual and the health care setting. Although it is predominantly ambulatory care, including care in the home, it also includes some types of care in the hospital. The number of people served per physician is smaller for primary care than for secondary and tertiary care. The latter two types of care represent consultative services in defined specialty segments, with emphasis generally on inpatient hospital care.

The concept of primary care bespeaks the continuing core of general health services. It covers, at a minimum, first contact, triage, full care of the more common illnesses and conditions, continued care of chronic illness, referral and follow-up for consultation and special procedures when needed, and preventive measures, including health maintenance and health promotion.

The paradoxes surrounding primary care are at least threefold. First, despite the policy direction of the past twenty years and the consensus on national needs, academic medicine does not accept the urgency of the primary care focus. Unlike the specialty disciplines, primary care still appears to the traditional medical faculty of specialists and subspecialists to lack a precisely defined body of knowledge for which special skills and training requirements can be readily established. Second, although many primary care functions can be performed effectively by nurses, physician extenders, and other nonphysician personel, the governance of academic medical centers, being medical faculty-dominated, prevents such transfers from readily occurring. New patterns of medical practice always develop slowly. They are accepted and diffused even more slowly. Finally, present methods and levels of payments to health providers for health care overwhelmingly favor inpatient and specialist care over primary care. Third-party payment agencies currently pay for over 90 percent of national expenditures for hospital services but only 60 percent of expenditures for physician services. Furthermore, the latter payments, based on "usual, customary, and reasonable" charges, are weighted heavily towards specific medical or surgical procedures.

Although the hospitals of the academic medical center are undoubtedly the most important resources for primary care in many metropolitan areas (in New York City these hospitals provide about one-third of all ambulatory care visits), adequate primary care can be provided by such hospitals only with major changes in financing, operations, and controls. In sum, the typical academic medical center is not currently set up to undertake primary care on a sigificant scale with optimum effectiveness and economy. Its refashioning will require action by both government and the centers.

At a conference held in 1971, commemorating the two hundredth anniversary of the founding of the New York Hospital, Alexander Heard commented:

There is no mystery about why in the contemporary American social and political environment, a medical school, teaching hospital, or university based medical center has difficulty and encounters controversy in defining its responsibilities. Starting with an acknowledged concern for illness or disability in individual American beings, there is a logical progression to and through all factors directly or indirectly affecting the health of that individual...Deciding where to draw the line is complicated by the genuine crush of objective, practical needs, by effective political and social pressures that are brought to bear by the quickened anxieties of many kinds of people, and by our mounting awareness of the interconnectedness of social institutions and of all human experience.[31]

In primary care the issue faced by the academic medical centers is how and to what extent they should serve all groups seeking care. While it is evident that centers should not be expected to assume responsibility for the operation of the total health care system, it is equally clear that society will reach out to them if adequate services and other institutions are not brought into being. Moreover, by the way they treat their patients, these centers shape the interests and skills of their graduates, and exercise a profound influence upon practice elsewhere in the system.

HEALTH PLANNING AND REGIONALIZATION

The academic medical centers must be active participants, even leaders, in the shaping of the community's health care system. They cannot remain aloof from the national, state, and local health planning processes. Here the questions are essentially those of resources, of costs and of supply, i.e., a deployment of facilities, technology, and manpower limited to the level required to furnish needed health services. These questions thus bring the centers face to face with the continuing issues of regionalization of high-cost services and the distribution of resources, as inevitably raised in health planning agencies. It cannot be said with confidence either that the present structures, created by government actions, are adequate to the task, or that the academic medical centers play the leadership role which, as university units, they should have the capacity to undertake in the interest of the community, region, and the state.

It is difficult to generalize about the relations between the 125 or more academic medical centers and the 200 Health Systems Agencies. Each center and health systems agency faces an extensive variety of local operational circumstances. But from the point of view of the academic medical centers, which clearly perceive the growth in external influences on their freedom of action as undesirable, the Health Systems Agency is high on the list of such influences. There is much uncertainty about the extent to which the missions and activities of academic medical centers should or will come under the planning surveillance of these agencies. It is not surprising, therefore, to find that academic medical centers, dominated by their goals in education and research, focus their efforts on "managing the HSA" so as to secure approval for what the center has already decided it wants.

On the other hand, because the Health Systems Agency tends to concentrate on the broad service needs of large areas, it often sees the teaching hospital first as just another hospital in the community and second as a high-cost hospital. Especially in an overbedded area, the referral function and special training needs of the teaching hospital may be ignored or minimized. This was, to give but one example, the framework for a recent prolonged and serious disagreement between the University of Chicago and the local HSA. Extensive discussions at the university led to further work by the academic medical center, including the faculty, with the local HSA. The overall effort brought about three salutary results. First, the university realized that active participation in local health planning was a necessity for the center. Second, the academic medical center came to realize its own need to clarify its mission, especially its service to the community, as it learned much more about its own patient load. Third, the HSA came to accept the character of the teaching hospital as an institution serving a broader area than the immediate local community.

Health planning had its historical beginnings in the requirement for state hospital plans mandated under the 1946 Hospital Construction Act, followed in the late 1950s and early 1960s by voluntary areawide or local facilities planning. As our health care system expanded, becoming both more complex and more accessible through enactment of federal financing legislation, there emerged in the middle 1960s the Comprehensive Health Planning Program (CHP) at state and local levels and the Regional Medical Programs for Heart Disease, Cancer, and Stroke (RMP). The academic medical centers showed only a pro forma interest in the CHP program with its strong governmental and consumer interest in services, but they were active in RMP, especially in the educational programs of its early years.

By the early 1970s, when Congress and the president shared a general perception that the health care system was largely out of control, health planning won further attention. The large and growing costs of care were accompanied by public concern over inappropriate utilization, excessive surgery, absence of consumer participation, and an apparent excess capacity of hospital beds. Congress saw at least an initial solution in abandoning the existing CHP, RMP, and other experimental federal programs for resource allocation and creating, instead, a national health planning system, with substantial elements of regulation. Under the new system, enacted as P.L. 93-641, the National Health Planning and Resources Development Act of 1974, Congress established that equal access to quality care at reasonable cost is a federal priority and that the management of resources to this end is essential to cost control. As overall guidance for the planning system at the federal, state, and area levels, a set of ten priorities was promulgated, starting with promotion of primary care, regionalization of health services, and prepaid health systems of care.

National guidelines issued by the Department of Health and Human Services include standards for the use of specified health services and hospital-bed-to-population ratios, as well as goals for systems of care. Through a tortuous series of compromises to accommodate diverse lobbies in the health field, Congress divided the planning function between state government agencies and local corporate bodies, whose public or private auspices were to be decided by local option. In addition, Congress initiated regulatory measures, such as programs of state certification of need for facilities to control the rate of capital investment, and state experiments to control hospital rates directly. Authority for this planning rests with a national network of some 200 Health Systems Agencies, which also have authority to review and approve, subject to federal review, hundreds of federally funded local projects.

In our introduction we spoke of the pluralistic essence of the American democracy and its manifestations in health care. The present national health planning system, providing representation by precise formulae and definitions to all special interests—providers and consumers, government and nongovernment, all levels of government—represents pluralism run riot. Unwilling to grasp the nettle inherent in resource allocation and regulation, but wanting to begin to rationalize and control the system, Congress has created a network of confused intentions and inadequate authority that leaves little opportunity for effective leadership, by academic medical centers or by any other group.

The effectiveness of the HSAs is severely limitated, although they are the heart of the planning structure where differing interests come together. HSAs have no direct authority to control utilization. Physicians' offices are beyond their mandatory purview. Above all, there are no formal links to the powerful incentives and disincentives of the health care reimbursement agencies, public or private. The greatest accomplishment of HSAs seems to be in providing an area for broad public

debate—or dispute—although in less complex regions, or where the
HSA and state agency functions are combined, stimulus has been given
to hospital mergers and expansion of needed ambulatory and home care
services.

The inevitable effect of the legislative mandate for broad representation of all special interests without provision for regulatory or
allocative powers is that consumers and providers alike tend to maintain the status quo within each HSA area. But because each HSA is
competing with others for available public funds, the agency is disinclin-
ed to reject proposals for new projects supported by such funds.

The academic medical center and its university associates in other
schools and departments can probably provide the greatest intellectual
resources for intelligent social and health planning. The present HSA
system has not provided an adequate vehicle for the expression of such
leadership nor have these university units shown much interest. Like
other providers, the centers look to their own special interest, and if
the system does not meet it, they are prepared to use other political
routes including direct contacts with state legislatures.

One case which received nationwide attention involved the approval
of a new hospital for the University of Michigan at Ann Arbor.[32]
Although the university had across-the-board agreement on the need
to replace its obsolete structure, it encountered widespread opposition
in the planning agencies. The primary reason appears to have been the
cost of the proposal, $311 million, which would have provided for 923
beds, 36 fewer than the present complement. Opposition was particularly strong in the Coalition for Health Care Costs, an active, concerned,
analytically sophisticated group of business, labor, and government officials, backed up by a state law calling for a reduction of 10 percent
in the number of beds in the state of Michigan.

After it was denied the $311 million plan and, subsequently, even a
$245 million plan, the university argued that the special role of a univer-
sity health science center was being ignored. Lobbying diligently with
the governor and influential members of the state legislative, it eventually secured the desired certificate of need for its modified $245 million
plan from the Department of Health. At the same time, for face-saving
reasons, it was required to secure subsequent approval from the local
planning agency.

The Michigan case illustrates two essential points about the relations
between the academic medical center and the field of health services
planning and health services costs. On the one hand, the exalted position of the academic medical center is a reality which gives it entrée
to the seats of political power. On the other hand, health care cost control and planning are also powerful political realities to which academic

centers will have to make effective adjustment and for which they are in a position to contribute mightily, especially through their university associates in other schools and departments.

Of course, the basic inquiry to be answered in all HSA planning is why every hospital should have the same services for all patients. The teaching hospital finds itself involved in two levels of competition with other hospitals. The first concerns the larger community hospital and its new capacity to perform consultative and inpatient services formerly reserved to the teaching hospital. This level is handled either by direct competition through enlarged faculty practices or through affiliation arrangements that stabilize patient referrals for both training and patient care.

The spreading responsibilities of the teaching hospital in this competitive process have had a subtle and not always welcome effect on the nonteaching hospital. The patient care capabilities of the teaching hospitals have slowly but steadily constricted or attempted to constrict the range of services provided by nonteaching hospitals and their medical staffs. At the same time, specialists settling with increasing frequency during the last decade in communities without a teaching hospital have wanted to practice the full range of what they had learned. In the absence of an openly adopted system of regionalization of services and facilities, the result was invidious resentment and unnecessary competitive waste.

Two contrary factors were often at work. On the one hand, the well-trained physician needs and uses the teaching hospital as a referral center when he believes that his own capacity and/or that of his usual hospital is unable to deal well with a particular problem. On the other hand, such a physician also prides himself on his skills and knowledge and gains special gratification when he can put them to use in his community hospital and not refer the patient to the teaching hospital. This factor is reinforced by the fee-for-service system which encourages expansion of a medical practice and perforce a physician's income.

Hence, a constant conflict, real or submerged, exists between the teaching and nonteaching hospitals and their medical staffs over the division of facilities and services. The conflict became especially obvious in the regional and other health planning processes of the late 1970s under the guidance of the Health Systems Agencies. It would become even sharper in a competitive environment in which provider income and interest, not public need and interest, would be the dominant considerations for service arrangements. Other countries, like Sweden and Britain, where quality of service is comparable with ours, have successfully addressed the role of tertiary-care institutions through regionalization programs under which the teaching hospital is integrated with community or district hospitals and primary care.

But equally critical is the second level of competition, namely that with the hospitals of other academic medical centers, especially in major metropolitan areas. We have detected a growing disagreement within medical center governance, especially between the lay trustees and medical professionals, over the long-standing effort of each major center to develop all high-cost tertiary care services and programs. This intercenter competition for prestige and power must be recognized in plans to regionalize high-cost services and in campaigns directed at cost containment and control. Because of the blending of education, research, and service objectives in the tertiary-care issues, these issues are rarely debated, and surely not resolved, within our health planning system.

It appears unlikely that the present planning system will last in its present form. It is too cumbersome, weak, and laden with documentation. In fact, the new administration in Washington has already proposed abandoning it, but Congress has only partially agreed. Surely, the policy debate will continue. Nevertheless, there is no doubt about the interconnection between financing of and eligibility for health care, reimbursement to providers, and planning for appropriate utilization and availability of services and resources. In view of the enormous public financing stake, we can be sure that these interconnections will increasingly force attention to the same issue that all of Western society has come to deal with—allocation of finite resources to deliver health services, whatever the needed level, for a defined population.[33]

However the planning issues are resolved and however public policy shifts between the extremes of regulation and of competition, the delivery of health services will command a continuing high level of public attention. Public finance will increasingly defray a critical portion of national health care costs in order to assure greater equity of access to modern health services and technology. Programs of the academic medical centers have now evolved so that their community service activities extend far beyond the level and type of patient care that they once deemed appropriate for the research university. Their existing activities serve not only community needs, particularly primary care, but also the concurrent training of specialists and provision of tertiary care, which have become the hallmark of the modern academic medical center. For these reasons as well as to create new revenue sources, the centers cannot escape undertaking large-scale service programs. These should be an integral part of any well-functioning and efficient health care system.

NOTES

1. *The Organization and Governance of Academic Health Centers*, Report of the Organiztion and Governance Project. Washington, D.C.: Association of Academic Health Centers, 1980, Vol. 2, p. 82.

2. C. E. Lewis, R. Fein, and D. Mechanic, *A Right to Health: The Problem of Access to Primary Medical Care*. New York: John Wiley and Sons, 1976.

3. American Public Health Association, *A Guide to Medical Care Administration*, Vol. 1, "Concepts and Principles," 1969 edition, p. 13.

4. *The Organization and Governance of Academic Health Centers*, Vol. 2, p. 5.

5. Robert M. Heyssel, "The Role of the Urban University Medical Center," in E. Ginzberg and A.M. Yohalem, eds, *The University Medical Center and the Metropolis*. New York: Josiah Macy, Jr. Foundation, 1974.

6. Irving J. Lewis, "Political Priorities and Controls: Implications for Medical Schools," *Perspectives in Biology and Medicine*, Vol. 16 (Winter 1973), pp. 280-286.

7. *The Organization and Governance of Academic Health Centers*, Vol. 3, pp. 39-40.

8. *Health, United States, 1979*, Washington, D.C.: U.S. Department of Health, Education and Welfare, DHEW Publication No. (PHS) 80-1232. Karen Davis and Cathy Schoen, *Health and the War on Poverty*. Washington, D.C.: Brookings Institution, 1978. *A New Survey on Access to Medical Care*, Special Report, Number One. Princeton: R. W. Johnson Foundation, 1978.

9. National Center for Health Services Research, *"Who Are the Uninsured?"* Data Preview 1 from the National Health Care Expenditure Study, Public Health Service, Department of Health and Human Services (Washington, D.C., 1980).

10. Louise B. Russell, "Medical Care," in Joseph A. Pechman, ed., *Setting National Priorities: Agenda for the 1980's*. Washington, D.C.: Brookings Institution, 1980, p. 181.

11. *A New Survey on Access to Medical Care*, pp. 11ff.

12. *Health, United States, 1979*, p. 8.

13. Association of American Medical Colleges, *Medical Practice Plans at U.S. Medical Schools*. Washington, D.C.: Department of Health, Education and Welfare, Health Resources Administration, 1977.

14. Robert Ebert, unpublished paper, "Academic Medicine in the 1980's—Optimism or Apprehension?" Winter 1980, p. 13.

15. J. A. Showstack, B. D. Blumberg, J. Schwartz, and S. A. Schroeder, "Fee-for-Service Physician Payment: Analysis of Current Methods and Their Development", *Inquiry*, Vol. XVI, No. 3 (Fall 1979), pp. 230-246.

16. Uwe Reinhardt, "The Future of Medical Enterprise: Perspectives on Resource Allocation in Socialized Markets," *Journal of Medical Education*, Vol. 55, No. 4 (April 1980), p. 32.

17. Russell, *op. cit.*, p. 189.

18. John H. Knowles, *The Teaching Hospital*. Cambridge: Harvard University Press, 1966, p. 104.

19. J. Feder, J. Holohan, and T. Marmor, eds., *National Health Insurance: Conflicting Goals and Policy Choices*. Washington, D.C.: The Urban Institute, 1980.

20. For a full summary of U.S. efforts at cost control, see J. F. Newman, W. B. Elliott, J. O. Gibbs, and H. C. Gift, "Attempts to Control Health Care Costs: the United States Experience," *Social Science and Medicine*, Vol. 13A (1979), pp. 529-540.

21. Rand Corporation, *Federal Manpower Legislation and the Academic Health Centers: An Interim Report*, prepared for the Department of Health, Education and Welfare, (R-1464-HEW). Santa Monica: Rand Corporation, April 1974, p. 88.

22. Robert Ebert, "Medical Education in the United States," in *Doing Better and Feeling Worse: Health in the United States. Daedalus,* Winter 1977.
23. Cecil G. Sheps, "Education for What? A Decalogue for Change," *Journal of the American Medical Association,* Vol. 238, No. 3 (July 18, 1977), p. 232.
24. Reported in Association of American Medical Colleges, *Weekly Report* No. 80-7, February 20, 1980.
25. Alain C. Enthoven, *Consumer-Choice Health Plan.* Reading: Addison-Wesley, 1980.
26. American Public Health Association, Community Health Planning Section, *Newsletter,* No. 80-1, January, 1980.
27. Daniel J. Fink, "Developing Marketing Strategies for University Teaching Hospitals," *Journal of Medical Education,* Vol. 55 (July 1980), pp. 574-579.
28. Robert M. Heyssel, "Competition and the Marketplace Approach to Containing the Cost of Medical Care." Unpublished paper.
29. U.S. Senate Committee on Labor and Human Resources, Report No. 96-936, "Health Professions Training and Distribution Act of 1980."
30. See Senate report above for past endorsements by the American Medical Association, the Association of American Medical Colleges, and the Institute of Medicine, as well as the committee itself. Also S. Andreopoulos, ed., *Primary Care: Where Medicine Fails,* a Sun Valley Forum report. New York: John Wiley and Sons, 1974.
31. *The Future Role of University-Based Metropolitan Medical Centers,* Proceedings of the New York Hospital Bicentennial Colloquium. New York: Josiah Macy, Jr. Foundation, 1972, p. 173.
32. "Michigan Outflanks Hospital Opponents," *New York Times,* October 4, 1979.
33. Bruce Vladeck, "Interest Group Representation and the HSAs: Health Planning and Political Theory," *American Journal of Public Health,* Vol. 67, No. 1 (January 1977), pp. 23-29.

Chapter 4

The Context and Conduct of
Medical Education

THE EDUCATION RESPONSIBILITIES
OF MEDICAL SCHOOLS

Among the major functions of the academic medical center, certainly one which is central to its social purpose, is that of carrying out manifold health professions educational programs to meet the needs of society. The major developments in American medical education in this century were outlined briefly in Chapter 2. In the light of public policy, these developments have produced great achievements as well as serious problems. In this chapter we first set forth in detail the evolution of medical education as well as the expectations of the academic medical center and its faculty, the medical profession, and the public. We then describe the expansion in responsibility, scope, and volume of the educational efforts and the predominant pattern of the curriculum and learning experiences provided. Finally, we examine the extent of match (or mismatch) between our educational programs and the needs of society, thereby assessing the manner in which the social contract between the medical education establishment and society is currently carried out.

Until the end of the first third of this century, medical schools had only one task, the preparation for and awarding of the M.D. degree to new physicians, who were then expected to practice on their own after obtaining the necessary medical license. Massive and multiple changes have taken place since then, not only in the educational program for medical students but also in the scale and nature of a diverse and growing number of additional training and education responsibilities which medical schools have undertaken. These new programs are directed both to the practice of medicine as such and to other health professions, technologies, and biomedical research. Consequently, the traditional function of undergraduate medical education is now only one of several major educational programs carried out by the medical school. Though formal responsibility for most of these programs rests with the medical school, almost all of them depend for their success upon the involvement and availability of other elements of the academic medical center. These programs are also continuously influenced, if not governed, by outside accreditation peer groups which review and accredit them. The expectations and standards of these peer groups represent the conventional wisdom of the day, embodying their view of the criteria leading to success. This gives them control over new approaches to medical education, its goals, and the methods used to achieve them.

While undergraduate medical education benefits in some important ways from the simultaneous conduct of other educational programs by the medical school, the effect is not always positive. Undergraduate medical education must compete with these other programs for attention, emphasis, and prestige. There can be little doubt that these diverse programs affect each other. For this reason, the size and nature of the nonmedical student education activities will be described briefly, followed by a similar discussion of the undergraduate medical education programs of our medical schools. Our medical schools differ sharply from schools of the other professions by virtue of the manifold and competing character of their educational responsibilities. In law, dentistry, architecture, and pharmacy, for example, the teaching responsibility of the faculty is concentrated on the preparation of their students for their formal, basic professional qualification.

In the two decades immediately following the Flexner report, medical schools concentrated on upgrading their educational efforts to prepare their students for the M.D. degree and subsequent licensing by the state. During this time, the larger hospitals, especially those affiliated with medical schools, organized their beds and services by specialty beyond that of surgery, leading to the recognition of most major specialties (internal medicine, obstetrics and gynecology, pediatrics and psychiatry). This aggregation of patients by specialties made it easier for the hospital and the specialists to concentrate, and hence enhance, their efforts in patient service, research, and teaching. In the course of time, however, it produced problems of fragmentation which have required special attention, not often meeting with notable success. The separation of services, while necessary and valuable, produced problems in integrating the care of patients as well as the education of students.

Most of the national specialty boards, founded to set standards of physician training for accreditation as specialists, were not set up until the 1930s and later. For obstetrics and gynecology the national board was approved in 1930, for pediatrics in 1933, for internal medicine in 1936, and for surgery in 1937. The larger hospitals established training programs to prepare specialists as their own responsibility. Even when the hospital was associated with a medical school, the school assumed no formal responsibility for such training. These programs were essentially apprenticeships, that is, the residents were given graded responsibilities, increasing in complexity over time, in the care of patients in the hospital who required the services of their specialty. The residents actually provided a large proportion of the direct medical services needed by patients in the hospitals. They carried out these patient care functions under a variable range of supervision by more senior trainees and the specialists who were the "attendings" in the hospital. Almost all of the latter group were in private practice, and only a small proportion of them had medical faculty appointments. Thus, in the early stages of its development, formal training for the specialties was accomplished almost entirely through programs of "learning by doing" in the hospitals where the specialties were being practiced. There was little other planned education content which might have brought them into the orbit of the medical schools.

In the 1930s, residency training programs began to undergo substantial change as the numbers of programs and training positions increased sharply. They came to be viewed as graduate educational programs involving learning requirements beyond vocational experience. Hence educational exercises of various types were introduced, supplementing and accompanying responsible participation by the residents in the delivery of specialist care to hospital patients. Included in these educational exercises were opportunities for research experience and for further instruction in the basic medical sciences.

Medical graduates came to believe that the participation of clinicians in the hospital who were members of a medical faculty brought a special and desirable quality to their postgraduate medical education, a term which then began to be used for this form of specialty training. This preference helped foster a trend of affiliation with medical schools which emerged clearly in the 1960s and has grown rapidly and steadily since then. In 1964-1965, for example, less than 50 percent of the programs offering graduate positions were associated with a medical school, whereas ten years later the proportion had risen to 91 percent. During this period also, as the drive toward specialization grew, the number of filled positions in all programs rose by 52 percent, from 40,894 to 62,236.[1] This number continued to rise, though at a slower rate, so that by 1979 it reached 64,615. In addition there were 4421 unfilled positions, largely in programs not affiliated with medical schools.[2] Thus specialty training, now known as graduate medical education, has become centered in hospitals affiliated with medical schools, whose faculty has assumed the dominant role in training for the specialties in medicine.

The association of the medical school with the hospitals that have residency programs takes a variety of forms, from close to loose. The costs are borne largely by hospital patient-care revenues, but some programs are entirely or partially financed by the medical school. Regardless of financing, program direction is centered in medical school department chairmen or training directors whom they appoint. Some affiliations involve an exchange of residents between the hospital and a medical school program, while others include only the provision by the medical school of educational exercises, such as grand rounds and seminars. It is important to note that the responsibility for graduate medical education rests with the various clinical departments and not in the medical school as an institution. It is rarely represented administratively at the institutional level, per se.

This large-scale development has had a profound effect upon the responsibilities, tasks, and activities of the medical school and its faculty. The magnitude of the direct day-to-day responsibility of medical schools for graduate medical education is indicated by the number of such residents for whom the schools see themselves as directly responsible. For the year 1979-1980 they reported their total direct teaching responsibilities as including 44,646 residents, as compared with 64,195 medical students. Some schools report having teaching responsibilities for a great many more residents than medical students. For example, the University of California at Los Angeles reported 1623 residents and 680 medical students, the University of Southern California 881 as compared with 586, and the Mount Sinai Medical School 848 and 454. Other schools reported a reverse relationship. The University of Rochester had 279 residents and 404 medical students, the University of North Carolina 301 and 644, the University of Texas at San Antonio 384 and 688, and the University of Vermont 155 and 334.[3]

Residency programs function on a day-to-day basis as an intimate component of patient care in the specialty wards and in the specialty clinics. Supervision of residents in the care of patients and the teaching-learning exercises of these programs engage a significant part of the faculty's time. They take great pride in the quality of residents they attract and judge their success as academic departments to a significant extent by this criterion. Furthermore, they join the residents in selecting patients for admission to their clinical service giving preference as far as possible to the types whom they consider to be most suitable for training purposes. Although residency programs are usually viewed as primarily serving educational and training purposes, whether or not they are conducted in affiliation with an academic medical center, it must be recognized that the residents carry the largest part of the burden of patient care in their departments as the essential and predominant framework of their learning opportunities.

A more recent development in graduate education has been fellowship programs in various clinical subspecialties. These provide advanced subspecialty training after the basic residency of three or more years in the specialty has been completed. With few exceptions they are offered in medical schools and funded through them. In the year 1978-1979, there were a total of 7178 graduate students in fields other than the basic sciences.[4] Funds to support these fellowships have come primarily from the National Institutes of Health and such national voluntary health organizations as the American Cancer Society and the American Heart Association. Some departments are also able to use departmental funds for this purpose. These programs, together with the residency programs in graduate medical education undertaken by medical schools, have had an important influence on priorities in these schools and on their ability to carry out their other responsibilities—an influence which will be discussed later in this chapter.

Another important group of full-time students taken on by medical schools are graduate students in the biomedical sciences—primarily the biological sciences whose fundamental relevance to medicine has been increasingly recognized throughout this century. They include physiology, biochemistry, anatomy, microbiology, pathology, and pharmacology. Although research and advanced training in these fields is also conducted in university loci and institutes independent of medical schools, in the United States and Canada graduate education in the biomedical sciences has been heavily concentrated in the basic science departments of our medical schools. The number of graduate students working formally toward a master's degree or a doctoral degree, or taking advanced training in a postdoctoral program, increased from 5166 in 1962-1963 to 8804 only five years later. In fifteen years the number had almost trebled, reaching over 15,000 by 1977-1978, and by 1979-1980, it was 16,704.[5] In addition, a sizable but unreported number of postdoctoral physicians are being trained on a full-time basis in these preclinical basic science departments. Just as the residency programs have added to and altered the mix of responsibilities of the clinical faculty of our medical schools, the great growth of formal graduate biomedical education programs has had the same effect upon the preclinical science departments.

This opportunity to strengthen and complement its research program by educating researchers is naturally very attractive to the faculty. It produces problems of priorities in their educational activities because it tends to downgrade their interest in "service" teaching to medical students. Altogether our medical schools reported formal continuous teaching responsibilities for 125,545 medical students, residents, and graduate students in the biomedical sciences in 1979-1980. Of these, 51.1 percent were medical students, 35.5 percent were residents, with the balance of 16,704 being graduate degree or postdoctoral students in the biomedical sciences.[6] In addition, many medical schools provide part of the formal education required for the completion of degree or certification requirements in other health and health-related professions. These include dentistry, nursing, pharmacy, and a growing group of allied health professions such as physiotherapy, laboratory technology, radiography, and speech and hearing. In such universitites, the medical school faculty provides varying amounts of organized teaching depending upon the nature of each field. The scale of these types of teaching responsibilities is indicated by the fact that, for the academic year 1979-1980, these types of students totaled over 63,000--fully half as many as the other groups of students described above.[7] Some medical schools also offer courses that are taken by undergraduate arts and sciences students in their university. Medical students make up only about one-third of the total number of students for whom the faculty of medical schools have significant, if not always complete, educational responsibility. Thus, the education program to qualify students for the M.D. degree is but one of a large and growing number of educational tasks assumed by the typical medical school.

Finally, medical schools are undertaking in increasing measure the continuing education of the practicing medical profession. They are now expected to do this, not only by way of leadership and demonstration, but also substantively in growing quantitative terms. Continuing education has, in the past fifteen years, assumed much larger importance than before as the question of maintaining competency of the practicing physician has become a subject of more discussion by the public as well as by the organized profession. As of 1980, twenty-six states and territories had enacted legislation requiring continuing medical education (CME) for registration for the license to practice medicine.

Many medical professional societies also now require CME for continued membership. Courses are offered by medical professional organizations, medical schools, voluntary health organizations, hospitals not affiliated with medical schools, and government agencies. As the academic medical centers have become the fountainhead of much of the new knowledge relevant to medical care, it is a natural extension of their mission that they should share, and thus help to implement, that new knowledge expeditiously and effectively among medical practitioners. Accordingly, medical schools have been expanding their programs of continuing education in recent years. Of the 2236 organizations that offered courses in 1979-1980, only 475 were accredited in July 1980 by the newly estabished Committee on Accreditation of Continuing Medical Education of the American Medical Association. The largest group was the professional societies, with 198, followed by 116 medical schools.[8] In 1978-1979, out of a total of 666 sponsors, 90 medical schools provided 36 percent of the courses in the whole country, an increase from 28 percent in the previous year.[9] There can be little doubt that medical schools will continue these efforts in the future and most probably on a larger scale.

The many different formal educational responsibilities of medical schools make it difficult for them to function with a central unity of purpose. Faculty members are divided in terms of their primary interests. Aside from their concentration and predominant commitment to research, of which more will be said later in this chapter, some are mainly interested in the education of residents, some in the training of researchers and some in undergraduate education. This diversity of major interests, plus the extensive range of sources and purposes of financial support available for medical faculty activities, is a major obstacle to the development of unifying missions of an institutional nature and to the establishment of educational priorities.

EXPANSION OF MEDICAL EDUCATION AND PUBLIC SUPPORT

We have already described the profound influence of the Flexner report of 1910 on medical schools and the education of medical students. The quality of medical education was improved by the infusion of the biomedical sciences, and the concept of the teaching hospital was adopted as the context of intensive supervised clinical experience and teaching. In the course of this process, virtually all medical schools were brought into the framework of our nation's universities. This facilitated the conduct of research and the improvement of teaching, as well as

the development of a predominantly scientific base for medical education. One important measure taken to strengthen these changes was
the gradual replacement by full-time faculty of the faculty who were
in private practice and taught on a part-time basis. This shift took place
first in the biological sciences and later in the clinical fields. The full-
time system which we now take for granted was given its initial impetus by the Rockefeller Foundation, which made grants available for
this purpose to several private medical schools in the years immediately
following the Flexner report. Not all were interested. Harvard University, for example, refused money for this purpose on the principle that
the care of private patients was an important part of its faculty's
academic life. Later, support for this change grew, especially from such
organizations as the American Society for Clinical Investigation, which
believed that faculty members needed to be free of the demands of
private practice in order to concentrate on developing and conducting
research and organizing the teaching of clinical subjects. In the course
of time, the movement to full-time clinical faculty became virtually
universal.

In accord with the expectations of those who supported the Flexner
report, the output of medical schools was sharply reduced. Within ten
years, the number of schools declined from 131 to 85 and the number
of students from 21,536 to 13,798. By 1930 the number of schools was
76 but the number of students had increased to 21,982. In that year
the number of graduates was 4735. In the depression years of the 1930s
there was little change. A speed-up in the education programs during
World War II brought the number of graduates to 5826 in 1946. In
the twenty-year period immediately after World War II, twelve medical
schools were established or converted from two-year to four-year programs. Eight of these were publicly owned. Before the war the medical
schools had been evenly divided between public and private sponsorship, but now state governments took on the primary responsibility
of creating new medical schools. In fact, since World War II only five
new private schools have been founded. By 1966, eighty-eight medical
schools were in operation, with 32,835 students, graduating 7574
students in that year.[10] Increasing state support for existing and new
medical schools continued through the 1970s.

Direct federal support for medical education came slowly, some time
after massive and ever-increasing federal support for biomedical
research in medical schools was well established. Among the many
government reports on physician education and supply since World War
II, a major analytic base for federal policy in support of increasing the
number of physicians was the report of the Surgeon General's Consultant Group on Medical Education issued in 1959. This document, known

as the Bane Report, described the problems arising from the rapid growth of population, the increase in the use of personal medical services, and the increase in the number of physicians required for new and rapidly developing specialized services.[11] As it turns out, the report overestimated the expected population increase. However, the cogency of the report's conclusions was greatly strengthened in the 1960s by the rising national concern to ensure equitable access to medical care for each citizen, regardless of ability to pay or geographic barrier. Major legislation adopted by Congress toward this end has been described in earlier chapters. It was assumed that more physicians were needed to provide the clinical care those legislative measures were designed to facilitate.

Direct financial support for medical education began in 1963 with the passage of the Health Professions Educational Assistance Act, under which the federal government provided funds for facility construction and for student scholarships and loans. After the passage of the Health Manpower Act of 1968, small operational grants were given to medical schools to increase their capacity to train the physicians to meet the nation's needs. The quid pro quo was the requirement that a school increase its enrollment by 2.5 percent. This was followed in 1971 by the Comprehensive Health Manpower Act, which for the first time provided a broad system of capitation grants as basic support to health profession schools for significant expansion in enrollment. The total amount available to a school was, however, calculated in terms of its total student enrollment as direct support for education. Bonuses were paid to medical schools that enlarged their entering classes above the required minimum of 5 percent, or ten students, whichever was greater, or that reduced the length of their curricula to three years. The medical schools saw fit to meet the requirements sufficiently that, in 1973-1974, they received an average of $2000 per student enrolled.[12]

The Comprehensive Health Manpower Act had another important feature—it overtly encouraged a new institutional responsibility for our medical schools in carrying out national health policy. A new program of Health Manpower Initiative Awards offered incentive grants and contracts for medical schools to develop programs not only to expand the supply of physicians, but to improve their distribution, efficiency, and effectiveness. Furthermore, to redress the widely recognized shortage of primary care physicians, it authorized financial support for the development of training programs in the newly emerging specialty of family medicine. This was very helpful to schools that had recently established training programs in family practice, a specialty which had first been nationally accredited just two years before. Moreover, the availability of this support for faculty salaries and related costs induced

other schools, especially the public schools, to develop such programs. Another program, created under this authority the following
year, was the Area Health Education Centers Program, whose purpose
was to improve the geographic distribution of physicians and other
health personnel through organized off-campus professional education
programs throughout the region served by a medical school. Although
most schools were not interested in this particular proposal, ten such
programs were started in 1972. Since then eleven others have been set
up. A number of these programs have also received support from state
governments, in some instances in very substantial amounts.

Federal policy shifted in 1976 with the passage of the Health Professions Educational Assistance Act. Although it continued capitation
grants, the law no longer required expanded enrollment. Instead, the
emphasis was placed upon the supply of primary-care practitioners and
correction of the imbalance in the geographic and specialty distribution of physicians. Thus this legislation authorized construction funds
for projects that emphasized ambulatory-care teaching and had linkages
with other federal initiatives such as family medicine and area health
education centers. It also required that, on a national level, 50 percent
of all first-year direct and affiliated residency positions had to be in
primary-care fields by the mid-1980s. Special project grants were also
authorized to improve the geographic and specialty distribution of
health personnel, such as expanded support for departments of family
medicine, new support for residencies and fellowships in internal
medicine and pediatrics as primary-care specialties, and support for
regional continuing education programs. Although interest varied
among the medical schools, most of them sought and obtained funds
for one or more of these types of projects.

By the late 1970s, a massive and unprecedented increase in the
number of medical students and graduates had taken place with the
financial support of the states and the federal government. The number
of schools increased sharply and the enrollment in existing schools was
boosted by expanding their facilities and faculty. By the fall of 1980,
124 four-year schools were fully or provisionally accredited, and two
schools conducted the first two years of the M.D. program. Medical
students totaled 64,195, twice the number in 1966.[13] The number of
graduates had also doubled in those fifteen years.

This expansion and the influx of foreign medical graduates led to a
46 percent increase in the number of physicians in active practice between 1960 and 1975. The secretary of the Department of Health, Education and Welfare estimated in 1978 that, by the year 1990, the supply
of physicians would increase by another 57 percent. He went on to say,

By virtually all accepted yardsticks, this portends a substantial oversupply of physicians on a national basis—an excess of 23,000 to 150,000
doctors by 1990, depending on how we measure physician need....I
recognize there are great variations, and indeed that is an important part
of the problem; but I am talking here about a national oversupply. Indeed we are already confronted in some areas with the consequences of
a physician oversupply.[14]

This perception, developed in the federal bureaucracy and elsewhere
in the late 1970s, led to repeated government policy statements announ-
cing the intent to abolish capitation payments as basic support for
medical education. This was finally accomplished in 1981.

The prediction of a surplus of physicians was set forth more specifically in the report of the Graduate Medical Education National Advisory
Committee (GMENAC) in the fall of 1980.[15] This expert committee had
been chartered by the Secretary of Health, Education and Welfare in
1976 "to make recommendations to the Secretary on the present and
future supply of and requirements for physicians, their specialty and
geographic distribution." The committee concluded that there would
probably be as many as 70,000 more physicians in 1990 than would
be needed. It predicted that the largest proportionate surpluses would
be in certain medical and pediatric subspecialties, various surgical
subspecialties, and obstetrics and gynecology. Also, it predicted shortages in such fields as child psychiatry, preventive medicine, and
emergency medicine. The committee made a number of recommendations, including decreases in admissions to medical schools and incentives to medical graduates to enter the under-supplied specialties. The
model used for its analyses embraces two components: current and projected physician *supply,* based on current training levels and projected
capacity, and medical *requirements,* including statistical calculations
of the need for various types of specialists to meet the medical care
needs of the nation's population.

The reactions to the GMENAC report have been mixed. There is more
overt agreement with the prediction of overall oversupply of physicians
than with predictions regarding oversupply in certain specialty fields.
At the same time, there appears to be more private and informal agreement among members of the subspecialty groups in which an oversupply is predicted than has been reflected in the official statements of their
national specialty societies.

Some policy changes will undoubtedly be made by government and
by the schools in recognition of the issues so sharply presented by this
committee. For example, in the *Annual Report of Medical Education
in the United States* published by the American Medical Association

in December 1980, Dr. C. H. Ruhe, its senior vice-president said,

> Although the major expansion of the medical education system initiated
> in the early 1960s had not yet exerted its maximum effect on total stu-
> dent enrollments, most institutions were already beginning to consider
> or to implement reductions in class size. Public perception was growing
> that the need for increased numbers of physicians had been satisfied....
> Emphasis of both federal and state governments has now switched to
> attempts to control the distribution of physicians and the nature of their
> function in the delivery of care.[15]

Thus the policies of medical schools regarding the size of their M.D.
programs will probably change as national and state policy change. In
adjusting the relative emphasis on postgraduate education for specific
specialties, they will perhaps be influenced much more by considerations of overall national need, as perceived outside the particular specialty, than has been the case heretofore.

THE CHANGING MEDICAL STUDENT

Over these years and particularly in the past decade or so, striking
changes have taken place in the types of students admitted by medical
schools. The attainment of a medical education has, in this century in
particular, been automatically awarded a great deal of public prestige.
Admission to medical school, while restricted to the upper echelon of
applicants in terms of demonstrated scholarly achievement and intellectual capacity, was also reserved, in the main, to those from upper-income
families. This restriction was due not only to the cost of medical education but also, for a time, to outright discrimination against first-and
second-generation immigrants, particularly those from eastern and
southern Europe, and against Jews, Catholics, and blacks. With the
expansion of medical schools after World War II, these types of
discrimination began to weaken. The most decisive changes, however,
occurred in the late 1960s, largely produced by three major social forces
external to the medical schools: the federal affirmative action programs
to expand the educational opportunities of minority groups, the massive
expansion of federal and state scholarship and loan programs to
facilitate professional education for those who could not otherwise afford it, and the women's liberation movement. Medical schools, like the
universities with which they are affiliated, whether publicly owned or
privately sponsored, came to be held publicly accountable for their performance in terms of these three issues. As John A. D. Cooper, full-

time president of the Association of American Medical Colleges, wrote in 1976, "Social pressures were brought to bear during the 1960s to increase the representation in medical schools of women, racial minorities and economically disadvantaged students.[17]

Clearly, significant progress has been made on these three fronts. For example, by 1969-1970, 58 percent of all medical students received loans to offset part of their expenses and 41 percent were awarded scholarships; 11 percent had received loans and 10 percent scholarships in 1957-1958.[18] Even more support of this sort became available in the 1970s.

Women have been a minority group in medicine for a long time. In 1955, they constituted only 5.5 percent of the medical student enrollment. However, only one-tenth as many female as male college graduates were applying for admission.[19] This low rate of female applications can be attributed largely to the popular visualization of medical school and medical practice as a "male world," to the inflexibility of requirements imposed on medical students and residents, and to the consequent lack of encouragement by college advisors and families. The rise and gathering strength of the feminist movement since the 1960s has changed this markedly. By 1969-1970, 3390 women were enrolled, constituting 9 percent of the total. Ten years later the number had risen to 16,315, representing a little over 25 percent of the total.[20]

During the same period an increasing number of schools took decisive action to begin to equalize the opportunity for entry into medicine by racial minorities such as blacks, Mexican-Americans, and others. To help overcome the typically severely disadvantaged background of many of these students, programs were developed to strengthen health professions advisory services in undergraduate colleges with predominantly black enrollments (originally with private foundation assistance pioneered by the Josiah Macy, Jr. Foundation); to institute vigorous recruitment and retention efforts for minority students, such as special guidance and tutoring after admission to medical school; and to facilitate the necessary advanced preparation and appointment of minority faculty members. In 1970, the Association of American Medical Colleges (AAMC) organized a task force to recommend a program of assistance to minorities. The report of this task force led to the adoption, that same year, by the AAMC's executive council, of a policy statement which, as reported by the association's president, "called for its constitutent members to direct earnest attention and effort toward the goal of expanding minority opportunities in medical service, teaching, and research. It established a short-term objective of 12 percent minority entrants by 1975-1976." This was double the proportion of such entering students in 1970. The goal was reached with the total number of students from all racial minority groups constituting 12.5 percent of the new entrants in 1974-1975.[21] While this represents progress, there is, in our view still more progress to be made.

The first significant rise in the enrollment of black Americans took place in 1969-1970, when 440 blacks entered medical school, representing 4.2 percent of the entering class—up from 266 (2.7 percent) the previous year. The number admitted continued to rise annually until 1974-1975, when it reached 1106 or 7.5 percent. During the 1970s, the total number of places in the entering classes rose each year. However, the number of black Americans admitted each year since the middle seventies has remained virtually the same, so that, in 1980-1981, black admissions represented only 6.6 percent of the entering class. The trend with Mexican-Americans has been much the same.[22] Suggested explanations for this standstill in progress for minority admissions include an erosion in the commitment to effective affirmative action and a decrease in availability of scholarship and loan funds in colleges and universities generally as well as in medical schools. Another factor is probably the standstill, if not retrogression, in the quality of public primary and secondary education, which is crucial to enlarging the pool of eligible students from the poor minority sections of our nation.

CHANGES IN THE MEDICAL CURRICULUM, SPECIALIZATION, AND INNOVATION

Medical education has changed profoundly in this century. Originally only a few years in a medical school were required preparation for practice. Today we have moved to the concept of a stepwise continuum of medical education to qualify physicians for practice by the M.D. degree, followed by a residency and continuing education. After the Flexner report the medical school curriculum became standardized and for almost fifty years remained quite inflexible. A minimum of two years of college education became an initial requirement for admission to medical school, but by 1930, nearly all schools required a bachelor's degree for admission. Courses in general biology, physics, general and organic chemistry, and sometimes German were premedical requirements. A graded curriculum of four academic years for the M.D. degree was implemented. Rigid examinations at the end of each year were the basis of promotion. The first two years were devoted almost entirely to the basic sciences, with much of the time spent in laboratory exercises. The first year laid the groundwork in anatomy, physiology, and biochemistry. The second year was devoted to the basis of disease and disorders, in terms of pathology, bacteriology, clinical pathology, and pharmacology, usually followed by a brief introduction to clinical practice through a course called physical diagnosis. The third and fourth years were devoted almost entirely to clinical clerkships in the teaching hospitals, mostly on the wards and, to a much smaller extent, in the outpatient department. In a series of rotations in different services such as medicine, surgery, pediatrics, and obstetrics and gynecology, students helped care for patients under close supervision of the resident staff and faculty. These clerkships constitute the first, and basic, foundation stones of the newly developing physician's clinical experience. They play a large and fundamental role in shaping his or her understanding of the tasks of clinical medicine and help set the pattern of later behavior in practice.

In time, the profession came to see the danger of rigidity and inflexibility resulting from the detailed specifications of curricula proposed by such bodies as the AAMC and the Council on Medical Education and Hospitals (CMEH) of the American Medical Association and then adopted by the Federation of State Medical Boards (FSMB), the licensing bodies. Some medical schools found some of the detailed requirements set by the state boards onerous and unnecessary. This led to a series of discussions among those groups as to their role in setting standards for medical education as distinct from assessing fitness for the practice of medicine. In 1930, the FSMB adopted a policy by which it recognized the AAMC as the "standardizing agency" for "all matters of premedical education, course of study, and education requirements for the degree of Doctor of Medicine," and stated further that the function of the FSMB was "a) the determining of fitness to practice and b) the enforcement of regulatory resources."[23] Making the medical schools themselves responsible for accreditation was seen by many as an important step in making diversity of programs possible. It led to the development of a cooperative arrangement, a dozen years later, by which the AAMC and the CMEH of the AMA joined together their complementary and duplicative efforts. The Liaison Committee on Medical Education (LCME), set up for this purpose, became the official accrediting agency in the nation for programs leading to the M.D. degree.

In the early part of this century it was still assumed that the M.D. program constituted sufficient preparation for the practice of medicine. As scientific knowledge grew and the scope of clinical practice broadened, it became steadily clearer that some additional training was advisable. This took the form of an internship, usually lasting one year and occasionally two. It consisted of a generalized experience in patient care in a hospital under the supervision of the attending staff in which the intern spent some time in each of the various clinical services. Some medical schools required the satisfactory completion of internship before granting of the degree. By 1930, the licensing boards of thirty states had adopted this requirement for licensing. Later it became universal.

As the medical specialties, after a slow start, developed vigorously in the 1930s, new clinical departments were established in medical schools and their teaching hospitals, each demanding time in the curriculum to expose students to its field. As discussed earlier, teaching hospitals were transformed into institutions predominantly interested in tertiary care. Their outpatient departments increasingly became a series of autonomous specialized clinics. These changes affected the content of medical education profoundly, both positively and negatively. They served the needs of the specialties per se, but made some wonder whether such institutions were really suitable as the sole locus of learning for the medical student.

Specialization became the order of the day for new graduates in medicine, producing a radical transformation in medical practice. The proportion of physicians in private practice who were full-time specialists grew from 36 percent in 1948 to 84 percent thirty years later.[24] The growth of postgraduate education for the growing number of specialties significantly altered the objectives of undergraduate medical education. Even with the internship added, undergraduate medical education could no longer be expected to provide full preparation for modern practice. The completion of a residency came to be seen as an essential requirement. Undergraduate medical education, therefore, came to be viewed as the broad base of preparation for specialization after graduation. This led to the adoption of the concept of a continuum of medical education after high school, progressing from premedical education to the M.D. program, followed by a residency of three to five years, in some selected cases even more.

After World War II several important modifications were made in the undergraduate medical curriculum. New subjects such as psychiatry and child development were introduced. The lecture method of teaching was superseded, to varying degrees, by self-learning under faculty guidance. Instead of rigidly prescribing the entire program in each of four years, schools now offered students some electives to meet their special interests, particularly after the first year. The major innovation in curriculum was developed by the Western Reserve School of Medicine in Cleveland with support from The Commonwealth Fund.[25] After several years of intensive and continuous study by its new, young faculty leadership, several basic concepts were adopted and implemented in 1952. These principles were: an integrated approach to normal human functioning and to the mechanisms of disease; the development of scientific critique; continued self-learning; and the cultivation of interpersonal as well as clinical skills. This approach called for much greater integration of teaching both between departments and between preclinical and clinical disciplines.

In implementing these principles, the Western Reserve faculty agreed to abolish traditional departmental courses—for its time a remarkable achievement in itself. Teaching by academic discipline was discarded, and the program was planned in detail by a series of interdepartmental committees. The four-year program was divided into three phases. The first year was devoted to normal structure, function, growth, and development presented in an integrated fashion by organ system. Contact with patients and families was established at the very beginning. The second phase of one and one-half years presented alterations of normal structure, function, growth, and development and the study of disease, also in an integrated fashion. The last year and a half was spent in application through clinical experience, with eight months of compulsory clerkships on the wards and in the outpatient department and six clinical electives. Student laboratories in each basic science department were abandoned. Instead, the students were assigned space in multidisciplinary laboratories for their own use; this home base was available to them at all hours. One comprehensive examination was given at the end of each year, graded on a pass/fail basis to decrease unnecessary and irrelevant competition among students. One and one-half days a week of unassigned time was provided, enabling each student to pursue his or her special interests.[26] It was clear that students found this curriculum more interesting and relevant than the orthodox alternative.

The radical changes wrought by Western Reserve had a pervasive impact on the other schools. Many schools adopted the program more or less as a whole. Others made their own adaptations of the basic concepts and procedures. Today, in virtually all schools, there is a good bit of elective time, generally equivalent to about one year. Self-learning under guidance has been widely adopted as a basic principle. Interdepartmental teaching in integrated blocks involving faculty from diverse preclinical and clinical departments is the prevailing pattern. Though there is diversity in detail, the principles and procedures introduced by the Western Reserve School of Medicine constitute the present norm throughout the nation.

Because preparation for medical practice now takes so long, interest has arisen in experimenting with the duration and content of the period between high school and the M.D. degree. In the early 1960s, a few schools introduced a program that integrated premedical and undergraduate medical education and reduced its duration from eight to six years after high school graduation. Talented high school students were admitted to these programs. Reports indicate that these specially selected students have done at least as well as the average in medical school, as measured by these schools. Whether these observations justify shortening the education program for all students is not clear. By 1980, 22 schools had adopted a combined, integrated college-medical school curriculum with a shortened time required after high school to obtain the M.D. degree. Perhaps because of these demonstrations, a growing number of medical schools have made arrangements to allow selected students to complete their full course of study in less than four years, largely by completing requirements during vacations. By 1980 this was the case in 43 schools.[27]

More recently, a special program was developed by The Commonwealth Fund to improve the interface between premedical and basic science training in the medical school. Seven private medical schools were given funds to develop such activities on a campuswide basis and bring the social sciences, the humanities, and the biological sciences in the university closer to the medical school and vice versa, for both students and faculty. It is still too early to evaluate the effects of this program.

RESEARCH AND MEDICAL EDUCATION

At this point it is necessary to examine the growth and role of research in the medical school, first in its own right, and second in its impact upon medical education and the other goals of the academic medical center. The exponential growth of the national effort in biomedical research following World War II, described in Chapters 1 and 2, has been the single most important influence upon the activities, priorities, curriculum, and governance of our medical schools. The volume and scope of this type of research has vastly increased in all developed nations; in North America, significantly, a much greater proportion of it is conducted by faculty within medical schools than in other university departments or special research institutes.

After 1910, the strengthening of biomedical departments such as anatomy, biochemistry, physiology, microbiology, and pathology encouraged the appointment of faculty members competent in these biological sciences and fostered research in these fields. This also helped to raise medicine to the level of a university discipline. It also fostered the use of laboratory-based instruction. Biomedical research in the first half of this century was relatively inexpensive. It was supported by the regular budget of the medical school, supplemented in the course of time by philanthropic foundations, led initially by the Rockefeller Foundation. By the 1920s, the leading medical schools were characterized by an increasingly scientific orientation that served as a model for the others to follow. This provided the basis for research during World War II and its further expansion afterwards. This expansion took place primarily and increasingly as a national effort led and financed, in the main, by the federal government, an effort already described in Chapter 1.

The nation's interest in research outgrew its capacity, in terms of suitably qualified scientific personnel and research facilities, and led to the institution of programs of research training, largely in the medical schools, supported by NIH. These programs not only trained personnel at the predoctoral and postdoctoral levels, but also led to the establishment of long-term support for selected researchers. These career research professorships were funded not only by the National Institutes of Health but also by such national voluntary bodies as the National Heart Association and the American Cancer Society.

In addition, the passage of the Health Research Facilities Construction Act of 1956 authorized matching funds, at 50 percent of cost, for the construction and equipping of research facilities in nonfederal institutions, mainly medical schools. Most of them were able to expand and improve their facilities by obtaining matching funds from state legislatures, foundations, and individual donors. This program remained in operation for about fifteen years.

Another significant program was the institution of general research grants, distributed in proportion to the size of the institution's research effort, available for essentially unrestricted use for salaries of research personnel, equipment, and seed money for research project development. Attention was also given to clinical research by providing support for special units in teaching hospitals known as "clinical research centers," where patients could remain for further study beyond the period ordinarily needed for their diagnosis and treatment without cost to themselves.

Only a brief indication of the scale of these efforts in biomedical research and the role of the federal government will be given here. For fiscal year 1977, the medical schools spent $940 million for research, 80 percent of which was derived from federal agencies, primarily NIH. This expenditure for research represented 23.9 percent of the schools' total expenditures as a group.[28] Of course, this ratio varies widely among the schools, with the more prestigious ones receiving much more than the mean amount for all the schools. Research constitutes the largest clearly discernible set of academic activities funded by bodies outside the university. In fiscal year 1979, schools reported research expenditures of $1.09 billion or 22 percent of their expenditures as a group for all purposes. Over the preceding twenty years, the total dollars spent in sponsored research had increased over ninefold. This represents a great proportionate growth in research activity within each school since, in this period, the number of medical schools increased by only 47 percent and medical students by 112 percent. At the same time the number of full-time faculty increased 350 percent.[29] The greatly expanded research effort conducted in medical schools is undoubtedly one of the major reasons for this growth in faculty size.

Starting in the early 1950s, when the national effort in biomedical research "took off," federal research funds were allocated each year in greatly increasing amounts. Often the budget recommended by the administration was significantly augmented by Congress. During this period, attempts made by the AAMC to obtain federal support for education per se were unsuccessful. Even though the funds appropriated for research were clearly earmarked for that purpose, faculty members conducting the research contributed in direct substantive ways to the educational programs of their medical schools. This was widely and openly recognized. Thus funds for research came to be viewed by the medical schools as support, at least in part, for other functions. This perception continued even after the federal government began direct support of medical education in 1963. Because research support became the dominant and most rapidly increasing source of funding for medical schools, it also became the hidden, and apparently accepted, subsidy for medical education. Hence the rigid approach to curriculum purpose and content, whose excellence and relevance the faculty assumed to be a function of the conduct of research itself.

The medical schools, like the scientific establishment generally, came to expect indefinitely continued real growth of government support for research. This was not to be, however. In the later 1960s, such funding began to plateau. In the late 1970s, the dollars available barely kept up with inflation, if that, and the prospect for maintaining current levels is not encouraging. Thus far, at any rate, this development has in no way diminished the dominant role of research in the value system of our medical schools.

There is no doubt whatever that our vast enterprise in biomedical research has produced new knowledge of great value in understanding health and disease and in the diagnosis, treatment, and prevention of disease. It is evident also that this new knowledge is increasing at a rapidly accelerating rate in many fields. Medical schools have undergone profound changes as they undertook to play the leading role in this national effort. It is not at all clear, however, that the resulting changes in how medical schools carry out their functions are all positive. The issues involved were summarized very well by John A. D. Cooper, president of the AAMC, in a recent volume, *Advances in American Medicine: Essays at the Bicentennial.*

> It is generally believed that the expanded biomedical research program enormously strengthened the medical school faculties and enhanced the quality of medical education. There are some, however, who hold that the unbalanced increase in research support has had detrimental effects on the schools; that it resulted in giving emphasis to research as the most important component of the medical school triad of responsibility for education, research and service; that the importance of teaching was deemphasized; and that there has been a subtle steering of students toward careers as specialists. Nevertheless, there is general agreement that without the research activities of the faculty, it would have been difficult to educate and train physicians to provide modern, scientifically based health care.[30]

While there can be little question about the validity of the general agreement described in the last sentence, it is significant that, in the past decade, the deleterious effects referred to by Cooper are now beginning to get attention from some prestigious figures in medical education as well as the general public and its representatives in state and federal government. Serious doubt is emerging as to whether the predominant interest of the faculty in research affects the education of medical students and residents in ways that help prepare them best for the patient care problems most of them will face in the communities in which they will practice.

Although there has been some leveling off of funding for biomedical research, it continues to assume a high public priority and national interest. Nevertheless, special attention needs to be given to the influence of this research effort, as currently organized, upon the continuum of medical education and the policy and operations of the academic medical center. In contrast to the Western European countries, where there has also been significant growth in biomedical research of high quality, the development of research capacity in the United States has been concentrated increasingly within the faculty of our medical schools. This concentration appears to be quite logical since the conduct of research can be expected to provide the elements of curiosity, the rigor of scientific inquiry, and the excitement of discovery which are essential ingredients of education of high quality in any field. Furthermore, the conduct of research helps to ensure that the medical faculty is on the frontier of new knowledge and can apply it readily in the care of patients, thus implementing and demonstrating its value without undue delay.

In the Western European countries, however, national research policy has continued to rely heavily on research institutes and centers. While many of these centers and institutes have some affiliation with a university and its medical school, they are distinct entities whose responsibilities are very clear. In Britain, for example, by far the largest single source of support for biomedical research is planned in broad terms and funded on behalf of the national government by the Medical Research Council (MRC). This agency differs from our National Institutes of Health and the National Science Foundation in the institutional arrangements that it fosters and supports for the conduct of research. While the MRC also supports research projects proposed by faculty members of Britain's medical schools, a very significant portion of the research it supports is conducted in units, centers, and institutes which it sets up and funds on a long-term basis. The members of these groups have no other obligations than to carry out their research. While many of these units are related to universities and medical schools, they are clearly and deliberately distinguishable from the university in a variety of important ways. The research staff is paid directly by the MRC. Though some of them hold faculty appointments, these are not the same type as those held by the academic faculty employed by the university. Their teaching is not obligatory and is generally related directly to their research interests and activities. Their work and their presence is of course viewed as being beneficial to the university and the medical school. However, they are not directly involved in policy decisions made by the faculty. The regular, policymaking members of the medical faculty are also expected to do research—and they do. In addition to research support from their university which is recommended by the national University Grants Committee, the faculty obtains support on a project basis from the MRC, private industry, and voluntary health agencies. Roughly the same pattern of organizing and supporting research is found in other Western European countries whose standards and productivity in biomedical research compare favorably with that of the United States.

In the United States, the freestanding research institution or center is the exception. We have very few. Research has, since World War II, been the largest single factor responsible for the substantial growth in numbers of medical faculty because our biomedical research efforts have been primarily concentrated there. Therefore, research capacity, proven or expected, became the single most crucial factor in evaluating the suitability of individuals for faculty appointment and promotion. Research productivity also became the single most important criterion used by medical educators in assessing their own institution and comparing it with others. It was assumed that there is always a direct positive relationship between the conduct of an increasing amount of productive research in a medical center and the quality of the education it provides. Moreover, while British research support is clearly for that purpose only, in the United States, it was openly accepted, especially in the 1950s and '60s, that this support would allow the researchers to give time to the performance of other faculty functions such as teaching and patient care. Thus the financial support for biomedical research served important additional functions as well as its ostensible objective.

This mixture of avowed and latent objectives clearly works against clarity of decision making about goals and priorities within the academic medical centers. Support for research from the federal government and other outside sources now represents roughly one-quarter of the budgets of our medical schools on the average, and all this research is performed by members of the faculty who have academic tenure or are striving for it. The impact of this upon recruiting faculty and maintaining them is clear and prominent. Especially at a time when national support for research is stable and perhaps decreasing, faculty members are under persistent pressure to compete successfully for continued and enlarged financial support.

The effect of research in the medical school has several aspects. Given the central and controlling role of research in the value system of medical faculty and its many different national peer groups, it is not uncommon for the discussion of patient-care problems with students and residents to place major emphasis on recent research which may or may not be applicable to the case at hand. In this context the care of the patient is not an end in itself but rather a means to the end of discussing the latest research findings. It is, of course, desirable that the evaluation and discussion of each patient should take into account the latest relevant scientific knowledge. The problem, however, is one of the emphasis of interest and the attitude this reflects toward the patient as a sick person. The faculty member whose status, prestige, and interests revolve primarily around research productivity must make a special effort in discussions with students and residents to subordinate those interests to the patient's overall health problems and needs. In addition, as already mentioned, research interests often affected the selection of patients for admission, thus skewing the range of medical problems with which students and residents are engaged.

There is yet another source of imbalance. The growth of postgraduate training programs to train researchers in the biomedical sciences has provided the faculty in the preclinical basic science departments with the opportunity "to reproduce themselves" as the clinical specialists do. The stimulus this provides to such faculty is, of course, much to be desired. The size and quality of such programs are usually the major basis upon which these departments assess themselves and are asessed by their peers. As suggested earlier in this chapter, the danger is the deprecation of the "service" role of the basic science departments in teaching medical students—a problem which has arisen in a number of medical schools.

Another common problem results from the fact that almost all faculty members feel strongly that they must concentrate as much of their efforts as possible upon their research. Their research effort is critical to their status on the faculty. In addition, outside support for their research often provides all or part of their salary and that of their close colleagues and assistants. Thus faculty members inevitably believe that their time for research must be jealously guarded, and tend to relegate the care of patients and the teaching of medical students and residents to a secondary position.

This dedication to research would be less important if it characterized a small, clearly designated proportion of faculty. The conventional formulation usually proclaimed by faculty leadership is, however, that all faculty members are equally interested in research, patient care, and teaching. The implication is that, with few exceptions, all faculty members of clinical departments are expected to behave that way. But the assumption of equal interest is highly unrealistic, and the bespoken interchangeability of roles has undesirable effects on faculty morale and on faculty performance in teaching and patient care. The fact is that most medical schools place major and controlling emphasis on research capacity and productivity in selecting individuals for faculty appointment and promotion.

The research efforts of our medical centers are overwhelmingly biomedical in nature. This work has been enormously productive and more is needed. As crucial as the biomedical approach to health and disease is, it implicitly treats human beings as if they were simply complex biological machines needing biological repair from time to time. But, the psychosocial component of human life also has a profound effect upon the health of individuals and groups and it, too, needs vigorous attention. Though this truth is rarely denied, social science research in health has been only minimally developed and then primarily in relation to mental health. The large role of social factors in health and disease generally has been ignored, as well as the crucial influence of attitude, life style, and behavior on health, and the ability and readiness of patients and their families to make adaptations appropriate to particular medical care and health maintenance situations. As a consequence of current research priorities medical education inevitably focuses predominately on the organic factors in health and disease processes in virtual isolation.

The foregoing discussion of problems in medical education which arise from the manner in which health-related research has been developed in the United States should not be interpreted as a lack of conviction about the positive contribution this research has made to medical education and medical care. The great progress made in biomedical research has provided new insight into the biological mechanisms of disease and has led to new modes of diagnosis and treatment. It has also fostered the development of new technology that adds precision to medical care and has opened up new areas of investigation. We believe that research is essential to the high quality of medical education and medical care required to meet society's needs. We have simply tried to outline some of the thorny problems that have emerged in the typical medical school—problems which need open-minded and imaginative attention if the programs of our academic medical centers are to be carried out in appropriate balance.

MEDICAL FACULTY, HOSPITALS, AND THE COMMUNITY

The activities of the medical faculty have important effects on the health service environment of many institutions and groups external to it, thus shaping their educational framework. These effects follow from what the faculty does and what it does not do. The most immediate and continuing effects, of course, are on the hospital(s) of the academic medical center itself. To a lesser degree, the affiliated hospitals not formally included in the academic medical center are also affected. The major affiliated hospitals see themselves primarily as central tertiary-care referral centers for their area, thus meeting the goals of the medical school and certain needs of the community at the same time. The question is how congruent the goals of the medical school and its affiliated hospitals are with the needs of the community. Even though these hospitals function as tertiary referral centers for the diagnosis and treatment of patients with complex problems that cannot be adequately treated elsewhere, all accept other cases as well. Since the affiliated hospitals are usually the largest, best equipped, and most fully staffed institutions in their area, they devote substantial efforts to the less complicated cases requiring secondary care. They also operate emergency services and provide a varying amount of primary care to ambulatory patients in their outpatient departments. (As discussed in Chapter 2, the demand for the latter services, while present everywhere, is most

marked in the urban ghettos in which many of the leading institutions
are located.) Specialists on the medical faculty are primarily interested
in treating and studying certain selected types of patients. The sum
total of these interests is rarely, if ever, fully representative of the health
care needs of the population, which naturally looks to the teaching
hospital as its major community health care resource.

The hospitals of the academic medical center have to face community expectations and demands much more directly and continuously than
do the many distinct groups of faculty members with their narrower
interest in their special fields. In addition, the hospital, for reasons of
fiscal viability usually provides a mix of tertiary, secondary, and
primary care services. Since secondary care is less intensive than tertiary care, it reduces the overall cost of care in the hospital. On the other
hand, when the hospital furnishes primary care to patients who cannot afford to pay or for whom the third-party payer such as Medicaid
pays less than the estimated cost, this produces an operating deficit
which has to be made up somehow. Given the current strong emphasis
on cost containment by governments and other third-party payers, the
need of hospitals to control their expenditures, and a national surplus
of acute care beds, hospitals are developing strategic plans for patient-
care programs that will embody a mix of tertiary, secondary, and
primary services allowing the hospitals to use their facilities fully, take
account of third-party payer requirements, and thus strengthen their
financial position.

Hospitals' efforts to "market" their services—the term used now by
hospital administrators—often lead to misunderstanding and conflict
with the faculty members who make up the medical staff of the teaching
hospitals. The latter generally tend to view certain health care problems
or patients as "uninteresting," not contributing directly to their
academic functions. Given the traditional goals and programs of the
academic medical center, conflicts of this type are to be expected. Accommodations between the two sets of pressures are sometimes possible. The medical faculty is more likely to accept the view of the teaching
hospital as a community health agency which must serve the community directly and remain fiscally viable when the hospital is a separate
institution governed by a community board. When the hospital is owned
by the university or is supported by the state government, the process
of accommodation usually takes much longer.

The pattern of patient care established in teaching hospitals affects
the physicians in practice and the nonteaching hospitals as well. In the
teaching hospitals the emphasis is upon the thoroughness of the "work-
up" of the patient. Involving a great deal of testing and measurement,
such work-ups often use more technology than many clinical experts

would think needed to make appropriate decisions about the diagnosis and management of the individual patient. The conventional wisdom in academia is that this approach is good for teaching because it emphasizes completeness and scientific precision, and that even when patently irrelevant, unnecessary, and wasteful, it represents the kind of mistakes students must be allowed to make as a learning exercise. This rationale, which was previously widely accepted, is now being questioned even within academic medical centers, but with little effect thus far. Faculty in the teaching hospitals tend to equate the traditional approach with "excellence," and it is within this framework that medical students and residents develop their concepts and habits of practice. Later they tend to function in the same manner; they expect, demand, and want to use the full range of procedures and techniques in the community hospitals where most of them subsequently practice. This raises costs for hospital and physician care without clearly adding commensurate benefits to their patients and the public. These habits of practice become deeply ingrained and have long term effects. Physicians would do better to heed the proverbial old Middle Eastern admonition, "When you hear the sound of hooves, think of horses, not zebras!"

A great problem in planning health services for populations is that the fragmentation of the service system can lead to the neglect of important health problems. A potential solution lies in converting individual elements of service into comprehensive programs of care. For hospitals in general, and for teaching in particular, this approach calls for extending their interests and services beyond or even in advance of the acute episode. Brilliant life-saving work for a patient with a chronic disease, for example, does little good if he is subsequently returned to the conditions of living and care in which his disease took hold and flourished. Typically, however, teaching-hospital staff do not see the development of such comprehensive care as pertinent to their teaching and research mission. Historically, as medical education developed since World War II, far too little attention has been paid to certain highly important problems producing premature death and great disability. Alcoholism and geriatrics are but two examples. Some programs of care and research in these and other fields have been started, generally with broad community support, but they are rarely in the mainstream of research, medical education, and medical care in our academic medical centers.

At this point, we turn our attention to certain aspects of physician development that are presenting relatively new challenges to our medical schools. From the public policy point of view, there are special problems in the role and responsibilities undertaken by the academic medical centers, individually and in sum, with regard to the number and types of physicians who are trained to meet current and future needs. As outlined briefly earlier in this chapter, comprehensive national planning to achieve these goals is at an early stage. It has consisted primarily of two types of efforts. In addition to providing financial support to increase the overall supply of physicians, special financing programs were introduced after World War II to increase the supply of certain types of specialists. In the 1950s there was a great growth in the interest in community mental health and psychiatric care. To expand specialty training in psychiatry, federal funds were provided for faculty support and for stipends to the M.D. trainees, with no subsequent service requirements. Later this type of support was also made available for postresidency subspecialty training in clinical fields such as cardiology and gastroenterology, among others. During the 1970s special federal allocations were made to stimulate and support training in primary care through departments of medicine and pediatrics and the establishment of departments of family medicine.

Long before these federal developments, it had been customary for state governments to establish and support medical schools mainly to fill the need for physicians in their state. In the postwar period, the shortage of physicians in rural and rapidly growing states was a major impetus for the rapid increase in the number of state-supported schools. Despite physician mobility, states found they could expect that about 40 percent of students enrolled in medical schools in their state of residence would eventually settle in their state. Some state schools have recently improved on this record. The medical school of the University of North Carolina at Chapel Hill, for example, achieved a level of 60 percent in the late 1970s.

In the past decade, the distribution of physicians by specialty and by location has commanded increasing public attention. The belief developed that a much higher proportion and number of primary-care physicians should be trained through residencies in family medicine, internal medicine, or pediatrics. Congress and state legislators felt that academic medical centers should try to channel more of their graduates into primary care. Some even expected the medical schools to induce a higher proportion of their graduates and residents to settle in smaller towns and rural areas. Except for a few recently founded institutions that explicitly emphasized education for primary care, medical schools were shocked by these expectations. Though academic medical centers were accustomed to competing nationally for federal funds to support postgraduate training in specialized fields, they were surprised to find government articulating national and state objectives in terms of numbers of type of practitioners and geographic location for practice. In effect, though the schools had been proclaiming that they were a national resource, they were stunned to be treated as such.

To be asked to tailor their programs to meet specific national or regional objectives seemed to the schools an unwarranted and dangerous interference with their prerogatives as educational institutions. The schools also argued that it was unreasonable to hold them responsible for the career decisions of their students, who were free to make their own decisions. But most students are known to be influenced by the example set by their teachers—what they do, what they stress, and what they deprecate or disdain. If primary care is low in prestige in the teaching hospital, as it generally is, if faculty members describe small-town and rural practice as inevitably limited, dull and of poor quality, then only the exceptionally insistent, dedicated (or benighted) student would deliberately pick those fields of work. As Plato has said, "What is honored in a country is cultivated there." It is worth noting that the small number of schools conducting area health education programs hope to achieve this objective, as do the community-based medical schools, which will be described later in this chapter.

MEDICAL EDUCATION—GOAL OR BY-PRODUCT?

The traditional core function of the medical school, undergraduate medical education, has to a significant extent been obscured by the development of the academic medical center with its broad range of activities, many of them carried out in isolation from others. Moreover, despite the presence of a three or four-year curriculum with a certain prescribed structure, the program of undergraduate medical education is typically not an integrated entity of its own. It is instead a by-product of many distinct, often unrelated activities serving the diverse objectives of a multitude of research projects and a large number of specialist activities and training programs. The assumption is that if these research and specialty clinical activities are of good quality, then it naturally follows that the program of medical education carried out by these same faculty members will also be good.

The medical faculty is not a coherent body. It is made up of groups and individuals with distinctive interests and commitments, whose strength is a function of their relative prestige and the amount of money available to them. The money comes from many different sources, much of it quite directly from outside agencies with special interests, rather than through an institutional budget allocation determined by the university or the medical school. The prestige of the faculty and school is largely dependent upon the judgment of their peers outside the institution, that is, researchers and clinical leaders from similar institutions who exercise their judgment on research and specialty-training grant applications. These peer judgments largely determine an individual's prestige within his own medical faculty as well. The medical faculty that does comparatively well by these judgements is assumed to be doing equally well in its medical education program. We believe, however, that this does not necessarily follow.

The task of undergraduate medical education is to provide the basic broad grounding of knowledge and attitudes relevant to health and disease and the major modes of evaluation and treatment of disease—all as a foundation for subsequent specialist training in one of several dozen specialist fields of practice ranging from family medicine, internal medicine, and pediatrics to ophthalmology, neurosurgery and pathology or in research. The assumption has been made that what the faculty does in research and in specialty care, when put together, will naturally provide the medical student with the full range of exposure, involvement and teaching which is need for his or her fundamental preparation for medical practice in the community. But the activities of the faculty, upon which they base their demonstrations and their teaching, were not designed with the needs of these students in mind. Hence the assumption that they can provide all that is needed for a balanced education program is unwarranted. In most academic medical centers, the diverse research and clinical interests of the faculty provide an intellectual smorgasbord that does not reflect many health problems that play a significant role in the lives of the public. The curriculum designed by such faculty is warped and uneven, with important elements entirely missing or referred to hastily and inadequately.

This problem has been clearly recognized in some European countries whose medical standards are comparable to ours, and is beginning to get some attention in the United States. In most of our medical schools, however, the educational program leading to the M.D. degree is a by-product of activities whose primary motivation has nothing to do with the basic education of future physicians. While this problem pertains particularly to the years of clinical teaching, it affects the teaching of the basic medical sciences as well. In a recent discussion of current beliefs and patterns in preparation for the study of clinical medicine, Carleton B. Chapman, M.D., then president of The Commonwealth Fund, said,

> The dictum that medicine has a scientific basis, and that the physician must be a scientist, is usually offered in support. But usually ignored is the fact that the scientific basis is largely a body of applicable bioscientific concepts, not a mass of pettifogging details. Yet most medical schools

seem content if the student masters the latter and have little concern for the former.[31]

Striking testimony along these lines was provided recently by Ludwig W. Eichna.[32] As chairman of the department of medicine at a medical school in New York City, he had found himself "increasingly dissatisfied with the course and results of medical school education." After his retirement in 1974, he enrolled as a full-time medical student in his school and completed the four-year degree program. He assessed his experience in a report he described as "largely a set of personal observations, reactions and conclusions ... It omits the good aspects, and there are many; it is more important to bring up deficiencies for correction than to dwell on positive qualities. Since the observations and conclusion are general, they do not always apply to all."

In the introductory section of his report, Eichna writes:

> Curricula, the basis of education, are devised by committees of faculty members according to their own concept of what is best, from their own outlook and at their level of knowledge. Each member contends, for the most part, for his own outlooks and disciplines. The most insistent usually prevail, whether they are right or not. Others yield for the sake of harmony. Too often the result is a patchwork, divorced from the essential purpose of the education.

The report subsequently sets forth some basic principles that should govern medical school education but at present are "routinely violated." Two of Eichna's principles deserve particular attention here.

Principle 1

The focus and first priority of medical school education is the patient.

> In practice, not so.
> Individual interests place their own desires and concepts first. The patient is too often a secondary consideration. The interests are vocal and insistent; the educational process surrenders to the principle. Medical school education is distorted from its primary purpose, care of the patient ... Faculty distorts the principle. Personal interests take over, and each member insists that a certain specialty receive favored treatment. A poptpourri results from attempts to satisfy everyone.

Principle 3

Learning is a thinking, problem-solving process that requires time.

> Medical school education today involves too little thinking and problem-

solving. It consists largely of too much fact and too little time, which is maldistributed to boot. The emphasis is on the accumulation of facts. Fact is king . . . Facts are essential. Problems cannot be solved without the sequential arrangement of facts. But in medicine the answer may not be there even after the facts are arranged. Students must learn to handle uncertainty; that too is medicine. Emphasis on facts does not teach them aspects of medicine any more than it teaches problem solving, and every patient presents a problem to be solved.

Ends and means have become confused. The task of educating medical students is rarely the principal consideration as faculty determine the nature and content of their activities outside the classroom. Yet these activities create the full framework and opportunity for the education program, which should be an end in itself, and not simply a by-product of other activities, however worthwhile. This issue in medical education is crucial to the future of health services in our nation. Studies have established that the experience of the medical students—what they are told, what they see being done, what gets the most attention and attracts the most prestige—has a profound influence upon their attitudes and behavior as practicing physicians. Education forms the individual—an effect well captured by the Spanish word for "graduate," *formado*, that is, the individual has been formed, shaped by his education.

The clinical framework used for medical student teaching, provides a good illustration of the way the education process has been determined by external influences. It has been assumed that the effectiveness and quality of medical education is directly related to the experience and teaching that students get in the tertiary-care hospital. The theory is that in learning how to diagnose and treat complicated, unusual cases of disease as well as acute episodes of illness, the student is well prepared to deal with the more frequent, "less interesting," problems including chronic conditions which are not acute, though disabling in varying degrees. This has become a dogma and it is almost heresy, in medical education circles, to question it. Evidence to back up this belief is hard to find. Although venerated in modern medicine, the scientific method has seldom been used in evaluating curriculum needs and effectiveness in medical education. For clinical departments and their specialized subunits, this absolute and fixed trust in the present program is a self-fulfilling prophecy. Its validity has, however, been questioned in other countries and steps have been taken to overcome its deficiencies. A small start is also being made in the United States, as we shall see later in this chapter.

THE MISMATCH BETWEEN TEACHING
AND THE PUBLIC NEED

The major problem in the quality and effectiveness of medical education stems from the mismatch between the health needs of the public and what is concentrated upon, demonstrated and taught in our academic medical centers. The educational program is dominated by the choices made in research and patient care, which reflect the interests of the many specialized individuals and groups that make up the faculty. Though each of these choices has some relevance to health and disease, when taken together, they rarely match the health needs of the population as a whole. Geriatrics and alcoholism, for example, present massive problems which get little, if any, attention in the academic medical center. The emphasis is on acute and unusual conditions, leaving chronic disease grossly neglected. The focus is generally on the unusual rather than the common problems. Prevention and rehabilitation are given lip service. Tertiary care is preferred over primary care. The patient in bed is deemed to be more interesting than the one who is ambulatory. The patients in the teaching hospital, where student experience is concentrated, represent a tiny fraction, less than 1 percent, of the total number of patients who seek medical care at any point in time.[33] How can this experience be thought to prepare students adequately for medical practice?

The neglect of important but "uninteresting" health problems in the educational program means that future physicians do not learn as much as is known about these areas. Moreover, little research is done on these problems, again because faculty interests lie elsewhere, so that progress toward improving the public's health is retarded.

The faculty tends to feel such criticisms ignore the depth and high quality of their performance in research, patient care, and hence, teaching. They point out that their students and residents emerge with much greater knowledge of disease and skill in diagnosis and treatment than did those of earlier generations. This we understand, accept, and appreciate. It is, however, beside the point addressed in these criticisms, namely that the educational program is not as well suited as it might be to health needs of the public. What is taught is what is best known and of greatest interest to the faculty, not what is needed as a preparation for practice. We are not arguing that the type of training now offered in the teaching hospitals is irrelevant but rather that students also need certain other important elements that now get little or no attention.

Recent graduates beginning practice often complain about these gaps and the imbalance in the curriculum. They find that they have been prepared inadequately or not at all for some of the important problems of care they face. Moreover, the reports they receive regarding patients they have referred to the tertiary teaching hospital often do not provide them with sufficient guidance in the further care of these patients.

The conviction has been growing that the currently typical framework of clinical education needs to be supplemented by other types of patients, not only those who have a substantial need for primary care. Some faculty members are beginning to come to this realization. In his 1980 Class Day address at the Harvard Medical School, for example, Professor Judah Folkman, said,

> You are fortunate to be entering the very best hospitals. You will be taught a myriad of new skills by the finest consultants and specialists, with the most modern equipment. . . .In fact, everything you need to apply your medical education to your future clinical work will now be taught to you, *except for one essential.* This essential is the most difficult thing to teach in a teaching hospital—*how to be a doctor.*[34]

He then described the price paid by patients and their families because of the fragmentation produced by specialized care as currently practiced in teaching hospitals, recommends that this problem urgently needs attention and goes on to say, "The idea that for each patient one doctor should have constant responsibility seems self-evident, yet, its actual practice is confounded by almost every tradition established in our modern medical centers..."

The public, too, shares in these perceptions. It finds a shortage of primary-care physicians—doctors who can see them readily, look after them continuously, refer them to specialists when necessary, and above all take an interest in understanding their problems, fears, and needs. This has led to widespread community demand for the production of more physicians trained for, and interested in, practicing primary care. Also, public organizations, governmental and voluntary, which concern themselves with health problems of the community, have been discouraged at the lack of interest of the academic medical centers in preparing their graduates to deal with such problems as health services for the aged, alcoholism, arthritis and other such health needs which cause substantial morbidity and social disorganization. The public appreciates the brilliant performance of our academic medical centers in selected cases. Nevertheless it is concerned about the mismatch between the overall thrust of these centers as they shape future medical care and the daily health needs of the public.

NEW CHALLENGES: PRIMARY CARE
AND GERIATRICS

These complaints about medical education have not been entirely ignored by our academic medical centers. They have begun to respond, generally in a grudging fashion, by offering new activities and programs or modifying existing programs. Unfortunately, with a few notable exceptions, these changes have had little effect on priorities among the major items on the agenda of the medical centers. While new institutions find it relatively easy to adopt a different set of priorities at the outset, as we shall see later in this chapter, they later have serious problems facing the pressures of the entrenched and prestigious status quo.

During the past decade ambulatory-care settings have been getting more attention as a context for preparing physicians for the tasks that will occupy a large part of their time in practice. Although the cogency of this approach was clearly demonstrated in a small number of prestigious institutions in the 1950s, it was not until the 1970s that our academic medical centers generally accepted the principle that the demonstration of high-quality ambulatory care was a worthwhile function. Before then, the work of the outpatient department was seen as a series of dull chores whose major functions were to feed the inpatient service and to follow up certain patients after treatment of their acute episode. Demands from the public for better conditions in the outpatient departments mounted in the late 1960s and thereafter added strength to the movement to improve the quality of institutional ambulatory care. These demands emerging from the consumer movement in health services and were supported by the new government payment programs adopted in 1965, Medicare and Medicaid, and by programs to organize new services.

At the same time, awareness was growing of the need to prepare physicians for primary care, which would clearly require turning more attention to ambulatory care. Some medical schools arranged for their students to gain supervised experience in the practice of physicians in the community as an undergraduate clerkship or as part of a residency program. Gradually, schools developed a more positive attitude towards ambulatory care as a professional function, and students, residents, and faculty became more involved in it. As a result, the facilities for ambulatory care and the delivery of the care itself have improved substantially.

The biological, social, and psychological problems presented by patients in the ambulatory setting, particularly those with chronic disease, are often more complex and difficult to deal with than those of patients on the inpatient service. Nevertheless, faculty still do not ordinarily treat ambulatory care with the respect accorded to inpatient care. But some progress, though slow and halting, has been real. In the clinical fields that have a large volume of patients such as medicine and pediatrics, most centers have now designated a faculty member as director of ambulatory care to supervise the overall organization and delivery of these services. This step is usually taken because the substantial growth in these services has created a need for continuous and consistent administrative attention. The director's influence on the quality of ambulatory care usually develops later and more slowly, if at all.

With over 80 percent of physicians trained for and seeking to spend full time in their specialties, the need for the generalist primary care physician has become increasingly obvious to the public. By now, most academic medical centers have undertaken to make all their students aware of this field and provide special residency programs for those physicians who want to specialize in it. More needs to be said at this point about the potential and problems of primary care education programs.

Primary care is the range of services needed by most people a large part of the time. The primary-care physician is one who is readily available to see individuals seeking care, makes decisions about what is needed, provides it or sees to it that it is provided appropriately, and gives continuing care during health and illness. When specialized care is needed, the primary-care physician serves as the patient's advocate and arranges and integrates the various aspects of the patient's care into an overall plan. This concept was developed out of the general practice traditon—a tradition which had long been declining as the specialties flourished.

Within the medical profession, some practitioners have been concerned about the primary-care gap for some time. Organized efforts to address this issue were represented by the establishment of the Section on General Practice in the American Medical Association in 1946 and the founding of the American Academy of General Practice the next year. The discussions stimulated by these groups and three major reports published in 1966-1967 crystallized the plans for action. These reports were sponsored by the American Medical Association.[35] the National Commission on Community Health Services organized by the National Health Council and the American Public Health Association[36] and the Council on Medical Education of the American Medical Association.[37] Each of these reports identified the need for "a personal physician," a "primary physician," or a "family physician." Notably absent from the sponsorship of these discussions and reports was the Association of American Medical Colleges, even though its executive director, Dr. Ward Darley, had gone on record in 1961 to declare the need for a "special kind of generalist who will need a special kind of training."[38] These efforts on the part of the practicing profession and those representing public and community interests culminated in the approval of the new discipline of family medicine as a medical specialty in 1969.

Graduate training in family medicine involves a three-year program, combining ambulatory-care training in a continuity-of-care setting with hospital-based training in the traditional specialties. At first, most of these residency programs were developed in community hospitals. Soon thereafter, responding to pressure and funds from the legislatures of some states and the availability of federal funds for this purpose, medical schools began to establish departments or divisions of family practice. Today 100 medical schools, roughly 80 percent of the total, provide role models, postgraduate training, and undergraduate education in family practice. About three-quarters of residency programs are now based in an academic medical center or in hospitals affiliated with one. Medical schools with such programs report that from 15 to 35 percent of their graduates enter family practice.[39] By 1979, with 6352 residents, family practice had become the third largest group, surpassed only by internal medicine with 16,580 and surgery with 7689 residents.[40] The residents in family medicine now constitute approximately 10 percent of the total number of residents in training.

Family physicians are not the only physicians who provide primary care in the United States today. Though they were trained to be specialists and act as consultants, many internists and pediatricians, as well as some other specialists, devote much of their actual practice to primary care. Controversy continues about whether these specialists are satisfied with this role or perform it as well or better than family physicians. A small number of the residency programs have recently begun to offer special "tracks" for those who want to prepare themselves specifically for "general internal medicine" or "general pediatrics." This stems from a deep conviction about the importance of this type of training and is a courageous departure from traditional departmental commitments to subspecialty training which bring the most prestige for the department. Charney has commented that these clinical disciplines have traditionally "focused on the complex rather than the routine, the diagnosis rather than the management, the acute rather than the chronic, the cure rather than prevention."[41]

A little tinkering with the traditional residency program in these two fields simply begs the question of appropriate training for primary care in these fields. Fundamental changes are needed. Clearly, family medicine has already estabished its credibility as a specialty with

medical graduates and the patients receiving primary care from its accredited practitioners. Within the other specialties, and especially in
internal medicine and pediatrics, family medicine is by no means fully
accepted as the best way to provide primary care in the future. This
view was cogently expressed recently by J. P. Geyman as follows:

> A general consensus has emerged that at least 50 percent of medical
> graduates should enter the primary care specialties of family practice,
> general internal medicine and general pediatrics. The federal goal for
> at least 50 percent of first year residency positions in medical schools
> and their affiliated hospitals appears to be met easily, especially
> because so many positions are in internal medicine. However, this gain
> is illusionary, since many of these primary care (general medicine and
> general pediatrics) residents will end up in the subspecialties.[42]

Geyman cites a recently published study which showed that, of a
group of 600 physicians trained in Massachusetts between 1967 and
1972, only 28 percent of former internal medicine residents and 56 percent of former pediatric residents spent more than half their current
time in primary care in 1976.[43] While some have argued that this so-
called hidden system of primary care will meet the nation's needs,[44] we
believe it has serious limitations.[45] Despite the substantial progress that
has been made, the best way to ensure a sufficient supply of adequately prepared physicians for primary care is, at present, by no means clear.
The medical faculties are unlikely to take this initiative in sharply reducing the size of their residency programs in internal medicine, pediatrics,
or other specialties. It is not yet clear how much of a contribution the
modified training programs in "general internal medicine" and "general
pediatrics" will make in developing primary-care physicians. Today the
federal government and most medical faculties assume that the typical
residency in these fields provides a satisfactory preparation for primary
care practice; their support has thus far protected this assumption from
objective testing.

Geriatrics, the care of the elderly, is another area that has been largely
avoided by our academic medical centers until very recently, despite
its importance to older people, their families, and society generally.
There are now more than 23 million Americans sixty-five years of age
or older. This age group, representing 11 percent of the population, requires more care than any other, because their age is accompanied by
the onset of chronic diseases and the greater incidence of cancer. Currently, the elderly use one-third of the inpatient services of the nation's
general hospitals. Although the importance of geriatrics has been
recognized by a few medical leaders for over forty years, medical schools

have shown little interest in giving this field, overt and continuous attention in terms of care, professional education, and research. Perhaps this is because most of the problems in geriatrics are complex, with prominent and crucial psychosocial components, and thus do not fit neatly into the categories of their faculty members' research and clinical interests.

Adequate geriatric care requires a complex set of biological and psychosocial approaches, the right cluster of skills and understandings at the right time, not more and not less. Restoring the metabolic balance of an older patient has only temporary value if everything else that needs to be done—medically, psychologically, and socially—is ignored when the patient returns to his environment. Geriatric care requires a type of teamwork and outreach that is not usual for our academic centers. They tend to believe that their efforts can be more fruitfully spent in other directions. Our present medical education system is aimed at cure, rather than caring and coping. While this orientation is understandable from some points of view, it is nevertheless unwise and socially unresponsive to the large-scale human problems that the field of geriatrics poses for medicine.

A few exemplary programs of geriatric care have been established in the United States. With one exception at most, none, until very recently, were developed in academic medical centers. The major deficits in this field were recognized first, and some time ago, by community social agencies, governments, and the public itself—not our academic medical centers. Several strong forces are now compelling attention to the need for large-scale positive developments in this field. These include a demographic imperative: by the year 2000, if the present trend continues, the number of people over sixty-five will be ten times greater than in 1900, while the U.S. population overall will have merely tripled. The elderly are expected to make up over 12 percent of the population, compared with 11 percent today. Moreover, the clinical and social problems of chronic disease and disability and the rising costs loom ever more imposing. The belief has been growing in the United States that everyone has a right to life with dignity and that steps should be taken to nurture and protect the capacities of older people. Some of these measures devolve on the helping professions and on institutions, and some on the individuals themselves and their own support systems. The tremendous change in public opinion with regard to the notion of a compulsory retirement age is just one indication of our citizens' new attitude toward themselves and their rights regardless of age.

We have lagged behind certain other countries in turning the attention of our education and health care system to geriatrics. In Britain, for example, the National Health Service was able, some time ago, to induce the medical schools to organize special efforts in geriatrics. By

1978, when there was only one chair of geriatrics in the United States, there were ten in Britain, a country with less than a quarter of our population. We have made some progress, however. Congressional interest, with little if any participation by the medical education establishment, culminated in the establishment, in 1974, of the National Institute on Aging to stimulate and support research on aging. Shortly thereafter the Student American Medical Asociation passed a resolution urging that geriatrics be given much more attention in the medical curriculum. The Ohio legislature gave serious consideration to demanding that geriatrics be included in the curriculum of the medical schools it was supporting. In large measure as a response to these external pressures, consensus is beginning to emerge among some medical educators that medical schools should develop strong programs directly focused on geriatrics.

In 1978 the Institute of Medicine issued a report urging that the problems of aging be given a great deal more attention in medical schools.[46] It argued that these issues should be addressed in the basic science and clinical courses, that there should be a required special course in geriatrics, that clinical clerkships and residents should also have this kind of experience and involvement, that geriatrics should be given attention in examinations, that students should work and learn in institutions such as nursing homes and other long-term care facilities, and that a faculty cadre with appropriate training for leadership in this field should be developed. The orientation of medical faculty towards this type of care is such that progress in implementing these recommendations will undoubtedly be slow, however.

In the late 1970s, funds for the establishment of geriatric centers for care, teaching, and research under academic medical center auspices became available from the federal government and, in some instances, from state legislatures. Some foundation funds are also now being offered for similar purposes. As a result of the external pressures and the availability of funds targeted for demonstrations of care, teaching and research in geriatrics several academic medical centers are beginning to set up programs to achieve these goals. To be most effective, such programs must compete with the more firmly entrenched activities in the centers and will require fundamental changes in faculty attitudes and priorities; thus progress will not come quickly. Continued monitoring of these programs by the external societal forces that have at last succeeded in getting some attention within the medical schools can help to maintain and strengthen these developments which are so badly needed.

COMMUNITY-BASED MEDICAL SCHOOLS

Chapter 2 briefly described the emergence of "community-based" academic medical centers. Departing from the Flexnerian model, these institutions base their programs of clinical experience and education in the community, rather than in a major hospital that the university owns or whose clinical services the medical school controls through the appointment of clinical faculty, constituting the hospital's medical staff. The potential for medical education in the community-based approach is different from that of the traditional academic medical center because secondary care plays a larger role in community hospitals, whereas tertiary care is clearly the dominant force in the classical university teaching hospital. Some medical schools have taken this approach as a matter of principle, believing that this is the way for them to achieve their major medical education goal—that is, to prepare physicians for their patient care role in the community. Other institutions have developed community-based programs largely because it did not appear to be feasible to build their own tertiary-care referral hospital or convert an existing hospital into such an institution.

The first and the best known of the community-based schools, the College of Human Medicine of Michigan State University at Lansing, was started in the early 1960s. Those who planned the school believed that basing its clinical activities within community hospitals was by far the best way to develop the new kind of physician required to meet health needs in the community. Other new schools that have chosen this path for the same reasons are Southern Illinois University, the University of North Dakota, and the clinical medical schools established at Peoria and Rockford by the University of Illinois as a consequence of recommendations adopted by the Illinois Board of Education in 1968. The Peoria School of Medicine was created by the action of the board of trustees of the University of Illinois in 1970. Four mandates for the School were enunciated:

1. To relate, whenever possible, the educational system to the system for the delivery of medical and health care;
2. To maintain its traditional concern for the undergraduate medical student, hopefully in untraditional ways;
3. To support, develop and extend the educational programs for house staff in the region; and
4. To develop meaningful programs for the continuing education of the practicing professional.[47]

Most of the community-based schools share these objectives, believing that this approach provides an excellent base for the education of physicians for practice. For example, a faculty member described the Primary Care Experience offered by the Rockford School of Medicine of the University of Illinois College of Medicine:

> The PCE program is conducted in these community health centers within a 35 mile radius of Rockford. The community health centers reflect the university's intent to operate the medical school as a community institution. Among the objectives of the program is that the patient, student, and faculty member engage in a dialogue pertinent to the delivery of comprehensive continuing and personal health care.[48]

The overriding emphasis on education and patient care in such centers does not mean that they take an adversarial attitude toward research. As insitutions, however, they value research in health and disease primarily for its contributions to the quality of their teaching, in addition to its being an end in itself.

There are now some eighteen community-based schools. Teaching programs in the community hospitals have been developed by a combination of methods. The hospital board and medical staff continue to have direct responsibility for the hospital's program of care. Full-time faculty are appointed to the medical staff of the hospital to develop and coordinate the education program; at the same time, qualified members of the medical staff practicing in the community are appointed to the faculty. Frequently, also, special ambulatory-care units, in the hospital or elsewhere, are developed by the medical faculty. Implementing such arrangements often raises some initital "town-gown" problems of autonomy of the hospital board and its medical staff, but these are generally resolved in a manner satisfactory to all concerned.   The College of Human Medicine of Michigan State University decided that its objective of emphasizing primary care and comprehensive medicine with a pervasive community orientation required it to develop new approaches to the teaching-learning process itself. This faculty pioneered in a number of ways. They gave the social sciences a much larger place in the scientific base along with the biomedical basic sciences, not only in the early years but also at the bedside, thus uniting human biology with human behavior. In a major curricular commitment to problem-based small group learning, they adopted an approach which they called "Focal Problems." John J. Jones and Peter O. Ways, both professors of medicine in that school, report:

> Since problem solving is a universal *modus operandi* in the medical profession, no matter what branch or specialty, it seemed appropriate to give

explicit attention to the development of the component skills of this process. In fact, the focus on the development of this skill was considered as essential as the learning of the specific detailed content of the basic and clinical sciences....It is our belief that Focal Problems has helped students to learn to problem solve and has exposed them during the preclinical years to a significant sample of the variety of problems (medical, social, psychological, economic) that impinge upon health and with which physicians must be concerned. It has provided a useful format for integrating and reinforcing content from a wide variety of disciplines. [49]

These objectives are not new and were identified earlier by other schools. What is distinctive and important in this school is the time and attention devoted to achieving them, the recruitment of faculty with appropriate knowledge and skills, and the learning framework that was developed, implemented, and modified after careful evaluation. A few other such new medical schools also took similar innovative approaches to the development of their curriculum.

Since the approach taken by these schools represents a distinct and radical departure from the well-established norm, it received little support or encouragement from most of the current leaders in medical education. Negative attitudes were expressed not only in private but also in the accreditation process. The open-minded scientific approach to the examination of evidence expected of medical faculty has been rarely evident in the attitude of the medical education establishment to this new development. Instead of focusing on the outcome, that is, the knowledge, skills, and demonstrated level of competence of the graduates of these schools, attention was riveted upon process, course content, and the facilities used. Any significant departure from the pattern of the traditional and prestigious academic medical centers was automatically deemed misguided and wrong, leading to the quick conclusion that these new schools could not possibly achieve their objectives at an acceptable level of quality. It was often seriously asked whether the objectives were not in themselves obstacles to the achievement of "quality." The main issues were the organization and teaching of the basic sciences, the role of research, and the absence of the classical university hospital. The new schools' emphasis on the social sciences as an essential component of the fundamental science base for the practice of medicine was perceived as reducing the amount of time that could be devoted to the biomedical sciences. But accepted ideas of the appropriate biomedical science content of a medical education are based on custom and traditions developed over the past half century. Objective evidence to validate the relevance of this content is not available.

A similar attitude has been taken towards the role of research. These new institutions certainly undertook to attract faculty who were interested in and capable of doing research. They accepted the crucial role of research on the part of faculty involved in medical education, as helping to assure an atmosphere of open-minded scientific inquiry and receptiveness to new ideas and knowledge. However, their plans and programs did not give research the predominant place it occupied in the traditional, more established schools.

A third issue pursued persistently by outside skeptics and in the accreditation process was the deep conviction that the university teaching hospital, fully controlled by the medical school, was critical to quality medical education and that its absence spelled disaster. It was assumed that the clinical experience needed by medical students for their basic education preparatory to residency training could simply not be supplied in the context of the community hospitals used by these new schools.

These perceptions of the community-based approach represent convictions held so deeply that experimental changes representing really fresh ideas were quickly and prematurely judged ill advised and doomed to failure. The innovations were criticized for the very fact of their clear departure from the norm without waiting for evidence regarding their effects. The new schools continue to encounter difficulties in the accrediting process simply because of what they do or do not do in terms of process and facilities. Although the only valid test is the quality and effectiveness of the performance of their graduates, most critics did not feel the need to wait for this evidence. This phenomenon has recently been described as a *system* problem by George F. Miller, the founding leader of American research in the goals and process of medical education. In the concluding chapter of his book *Educating Medical Teachers,* he says:

> Turning first to *system problems,* few observers would deny that medical faculties are dominated by basic and clinical scientists whose first loyalty is advancement of the discipline with which they are identified. However, any dispassionate analyst would also acknowledge that a faculty member really has two disciplines—one biomedical, the other educational. Yet the spirit of scientific inquiry, which should characterize both, seems generally to be left in the laboratory when it is time to move to the classroom. Curiously, this discrepancy is rarely recognized and even less frequently verbalized. Scientists who refuse to accept Krebiozen or Laetrile on the basis of testimonials see nothing strange about embracing methods of instruction and evaluation whose use is supported by nothing more substantial. Investigators who insist that systematic study of biologic phenomena, rather than individual experience, must be the base from

which to draw conclusions see nothing inconsistent in any rejection of carefully planned educational studies whose findings fail to match their personal preferences. Medical teachers seem quite prepared to accept data that support the educational views they hold but are strangely unresponsive to findings that suggest a need for change in the way they do things. Arrogance may be too strong a word to describe this behavior, but it is certainly closer to reality than the spirit of inquiry that is always claimed as the hallmark of higher professional education.[50]

Despite these pressures, the community-based schools have persisted, although some have submitted to the pressures and modified their programs substantially, thus reverting to the mainstream to varying degrees. By now, a few cohorts of community-based medical school graduates have completed their residencies and gone into practice. The indications are that, as a group, they compare favorably with the graduates of the traditional schools. Certainly there is no clear evidence to support the dire predictions of their critics. Of course, it will take perhaps another decade before rigorous systematic studies can be made of the differences between the graduates of these schools and others. There can now be little doubt, however, that the community-based approach has merit.

THE STALEMATE OF SUCCESS

David Riesman, in writing of education in America, has described the phenomenon of the "stalemate of success."[51] The concept has particular relevance for medical education today. The radical changes in medical education that followed the Flexner report were vast improvements. The move to the university, the emphasis on the science base, and the development of full-time faculty for clinical as well as basic science teaching and research put medical schools in a sound position to participate in the explosion of scientific research that came mainly after World War II by medical schools expanding into major biomedical research centers. The rapidly accelerating accumulation of new knowledge inevitably also led to increasing specialization and subspecialization in medical practice. Medical faculties grew prodigiously in size in order to carry out research, mainly in the biomedical sciences, and to add a broad spectrum of postgraduate specialty training programs in established as well as in newly emerging fields. These twin developments became the strongest movements within academic medical centers. Favorable peer review of such specialized activities became the major source of prestige and acclaim. As a consequence, research and specialty training also brought additional funds to the institution for the specific use of designated faculty members who had successfully applied for them.

Research and the development of new technology have flourished. More always remained to be done to improve our knowledge of the causes, diagnosis, and treatment of the disease entities chosen for study. Altogether, this has been a story of brilliant successes, especially in the eyes of the faculty—new knowledge, new specialization, and prestige and recognition by peers and the general public. It was perhaps natural for faculties to assume that their undergraduate medical education programs were of similar high quality, since they were a direct reflection of their research and specialty training programs. Implicit is the assumption that the best approach to education is simply to sum the specific goals and activities of each faculty unit. Consequently it seems obvious that any need for improvement can best be met by doing more of the same. Hence the stalemate of success—a single-minded approach only.

Changes in the emphasis and process of education are often viewed as misguided or even subversive. Individual faculty members prefer not to risk radically new ventures, when the road to success has been so clearly demonstrated to them in the past quarter-century. Prestigious, successful faculty leaders in medicine, as in all fields, are not noted for welcoming new goals or criteria different from those that brought success to them. Instead, they prefer to intensify their efforts incrementally in fields of work that are considered prestigious and well accepted by their professional peer group. The readiness to be daring and take risks in concept and method, which characterizes of the best of scientific research, is rarely encountered in people asked to evaluate the relevance of their work to other fields, in this case with reference to medical education. Thus, faculty members prefer to ignore the pressures for more attention to ambulatory care, primary care, geriatrics, or alcoholism, because they see plenty of unexploited potential in what they are already doing. Continued pressures often elicit only a token response, with the faculty doing as much as necessary but as little as possible. As a result, the service, teaching, and research activities undertaken to meet changing societal health needs are generally at the periphery of the academic medical center's interests rather than at its core, and rarely compete successfully with all the traditional, entrenched faculty interests.

By constricting the scope, strength, and effectiveness of the academic center in meeting certain vital needs in community health, these attitudes produce educational and training deficits in fields beyond the medical profession as well as within it. As we have pointed out before, other health professions are dependent in crucial ways upon the priorities, the pattern, and the restricted framework of patient care in the academic medical center. The center determines the types of care that are welcomed or spurned and thus frames and controls the opportunities and priorities in the education of nurses, dentists, pharmacists, social workers, and health educators. These professions have identified as critical health needs such areas as chronic disease, geriatrics, ambulatory care, health maintenance, and disease prevention. Long ago, for example, nursing educators began to respond to the geriatric nursing needs in the community by developing special programs of continued education and giving these problems more attention in their undergraduate nursing teaching programs. They could demonstrate little indeed within their own medical centers, however, because of the lack of interest of the medical faculty. Long-term care presents important challenges to nursing, social work, and physical and vocational therapy, as well as to medicine, to devise effective team care programs for these patients, who number in the millions. In 1977, for example, there were 1.3 million people in nursing homes, of whom 86.4 percent were sixty-five years of age or older.[52] How can long-term care and the rapidly growing nursing home segment of our health system be explored, tested, and improved if the major institutional and professional discipline of medicine is not interested in it and does not work close in it with the other health professions in patient care, education, and research? Without this, how can we develop the restorative potential of many of the patients in long-term care? This exemplifies a most serious and pressing question to which the academic medical center provides no answer and in which it shows small interest.

NEEDED REFORMS

This chapter has tried to provide an understanding of today's achievements and challenges in medical education by describing its evolution, its present orientation, scope and emphasis, the forces that currently control it, the problems of change, and the resulting effects upon the health services system of our nation. Borrowing the metaphor used by E. M. Forster in his famous essay on democracy, we give two cheers for our medical education system. Like Forster, we withhold the third cheer because we believe that certain crucial elements are missing, elements needed if our academic medical centers are to fulfill adequately the needs and expectations of our society for the improvement of health care. This is the crux of the social contract between the academic medical centers and the public which supports them.

We conclude that medical education, and especially that leading to the M.D. degree, needs radical reform. Undergraduate medical education is now largely a by-product of a large series of discrete research and clinical care activities undertaken without sufficient regard to their direct relevance to the educational task. This deficiency needs to be repaired. Adding a few new activities at the periphery will not be sufficient; rather, all the priorities of the academic medical center must be reordered to meet educational and community health needs. The problems in postgraduate medical education have to do with establishing guidelines for the types and numbers of specialists that should be trained to meet national needs and inculcating an evaluative approach to the appropriate use of technology in patient care.

Research opportunities will not be diminished by these changes. They will lead to new frontiers of research and patient care that need to be broached. The major thrust of twentieth-century academic medicine in biomedical research and specialization, which reinforce each other though creating some problems for us now, has brought great benefits to society. It has led to brilliant discoveries regarding the origin and development of some disease conditions. It has developed brilliant technology which, though sometimes misused, is nevertheless crucial to diagnosis and treatment in properly selected cases. It has produced preventive measures such as immunizations and remedial treatment such as antibiotics, hip joint replacements, and cardiac surgery. Clearly, there is much to be grateful for. However, as one of us said some years ago,

> These developments have brought great benefits. They have also exacted a price. It is what they have displaced, neglected, or overdone that contributes substantially to the present dissatisfactions with medical care and medical education.... The overemphasis on tertiary care in the university medical centers distorts their educational programs. The fixation on the disease concept of illness in biological terms only, is an inadequate, inappropriate, and skewed preparation for the care of most patients in the community. Patient care is no longer coincident with the power to prescribe because health-care problems and opportunities are augmented by many aspects of human life.[53]

This latter point applies strongly to the most prevalent and chronic health problems of people, although it may be less critical in the acute episode that requires hospitalization. The emphasis in medical education on the biomedical sciences, specialization, and technology has given physicians a strong sense of the value of their work. At the same time, however, it has produced a kind of professional isolation that is more suitable for the research laboratory than for the practice of human medicine. It makes no sense to separate human health and disease from the human being and the environment in which people live. The scientific approach requires the evaluation of *all* the facts that operate in the system addressed by a specific inquiry. To collect and evaluate a large series of physiochemical facts about a person and not match them with relevant social, psychological, and economic facts is to be incomplete as well as unscientific. While this full range of fact gathering and assessment is less crucial, at least initially, in the case of a broken leg or a perforated stomach ulcer, it is fundamental to optimal care with the large majority of chronic illnesses, in maternal and child health, geriatrics, and occupational disease, to name but a few.

It must be recognized that medicine as a profession has a continuing and vital sustaining function that cannot be carried out by the application of biomedical technology alone. It is simply inadequate to take the stand, as some leaders in academic medicine do, that physicians can view illness simply as deranged biomedical function.[54] Unless our academic medical centers broaden the base of their activities and interests to give psychosocial elements as much continuing attention as is now given to biological aspects, medicine's crisis and public disappointment and chagrin will continue and deepen.

Another fundamental reform needed is to recognize the severe limitations of the highly selective scope of care that now serves as the context of medical education. This range of services, which has been determined largely by the research and specialty practice interests of the faculty in an inner-directed way, results in a profound mismatch between what is taught and what is needed to serve public and individual health goals. To correct this imbalance, the academic medical center must take responsibility for the delivery of the full range of medical care so that, while carrying out its tertiary-care functions, it also gives creative attention to primary and secondary care and the optimum relationship between all three levels. In rendering these services and education programs, the centers should be directly responsive to community needs, as seen from the epidemiological point of view, that is, the community as a whole. They must become involved in the full range of health problems of their region. Our academic medical centers should play a leading role in building a comprehensive program of medical care to meet the needs of their regions in an effective, balanced, and economical manner: this effort should provide the major context for teaching and learning in medical and other health professions education.

NOTES

1. Association of American Medical Colleges, *Medical Education: Institutions, Characteristics and Programs* (Washington, D. C., 1979), p. 5, p. 17, Figure 16.
2. "Medical Education in the United States, 1979-1980," *Journal of the American Medical Association*, Vol. 244, No. 25 (Dec. 26, 1980), p. 2830, Table 4; p. 2829, Table 2.
3. *Ibid.*, pp. 2853-2855, Appendix II, Table 3.
4. *Ibid.*, p. 2811.
5. Association of American Medical Colleges, *op. cit.*, p. 12, Figure 3.
6. "Medical Education in the United States, 1979-1980," *op. cit.*, p. 2855.
7. *Ibid.*, p. 2811.
8. *Ibid.*, p. 2837, Table 5.
9. *Ibid.*, p. 2837, Table 6. "Medical Education in the United States, 1978-79," *Journal of the American Medical Association*, Vol. 243, No. 9 (March 7, 1980) p. 895, Table 12.
10. C. G. Sheps and C. Seipp, "The Medical School, Its Products and Its Problems," *Annals of American Association of Political Science*, Vol. 399, No. 43 (Jan. 1972).
11. C. C. Fordham, "The Bane Report Revisited," *Journal of the American Medical Association*, Vol. 244, No. 4, (July 27, 1980), pp. 354-357.
12. J. A. D. Cooper, in J. Z. Bowers and E. F. Purcell, *Advances in American Medicine: Essays at the Bicentennial.* (New York: Josiah Macy, Jr. Foundation, 1976), Vol. I, p. 295.
13. "Medical Education in the United States, 1979-1980," *op. cit.* p. 2810, Table 1.
14. J. A. Califano, "The Government—Medical Education Partnership," *Journal of Medical Education*, Vol. 54 (Jan. 1979), pp. 19-20.
15. Graduate Medical Education National Advisory Committee, "Report to the Secretary, Department of Health and Human Services," September 1980.
16. C. H. Ruhe, "Recent Events of Special Interest to Medical Education," *Journal of the American Medical Association*, Vol. 244, No. 25 (Dec. 26, 1980), p. 2805.
17. Cooper, *op. cit.*, p. 281.
18. Sheps and Seipp, *op. cit.*, pp. 44-45.
19. *Ibid.*
20. "Medical Education in the United States, 1979-1980," *op. cit.*, p. 2814, Table 10.
21. Cooper, *op. cit.*, pp. 282-283.
22. Association of American Medical Colleges, "Medical School Admission Requirements 1981-82," "1980-81 Fall Enrollment Survey," "1971-76 Enrollment Survey."
23. Commission on Medical Education, *Medical Education: Final Report of the Commission on Medical Education.* (New York, 1932), Vol. 1, p. 167.
24. A. Donabedian, S. J. Axelrod, and L. Wyszewianski, *Medical Care Chart Book.* (Ann Arbor: AUPHA Press, 1980), p. 159.
25. G. Williams, *Western Reserve's Experiment in Medical Education and Its Outcome.* (New York: Oxford University Press, 1980).
26. Cooper, *op. cit.*, pp. 284-285.
27. "Medical Education in the United States, 1979-1980," *op. cit.*, p. 2817.
28. Association of American Medical Colleges, *Medical Education:* p. 7, p. 18, Figure 20.
29. "Medical Education in the United States, 1979-1980," *op. cit.*, p. 2819, Table 24.
30. Cooper, *op. cit.*, p. 276.
31. C. B. Chapman, "Should There Be a Commission on Medical Education?" *Science*, Vol. 205 (Aug. 10, 1979), p. 561.
32. L. W. Eichna, "Medical School Education, 1975-79," *New England Journal of Medicine*, Vol. 303, No. 13 (Sept. 25, 1980), pp. 227-234.

33. K. L. White, T. F. Williams, and B. G. Greenberg, "The Ecology of Medical Care," *New England Journal of Medicine*, Vol. 265 (Nov. 2, 1961), pp. 885-892.

34. J. Falkman, "Is There a Doctor in the House?" *Harvard Medical Alumni Bulletin*, Vol. 54, No. 5 (Aug. 1980), pp. 37-40.

35. J. Millis, *The Graduate Education of Physicians*. Report of the Citizens' Commission on Graduate Medical Education. (Chicago: American Medical Association, 1966).

36. *Health is a Community Affair*. (Cambridge, Mass.: Harvard University Press, 1967), pp. 202, 205.

37. W. R. Willard, *Meeting the Challenge of Family Practice*. (Chicago: American Medical Association), pp. 14, 37.

38. W. Darley, "Response, Concerns, Encouragements and Hopes for Comprehensive Medicine," *Journal of Medical Education*, Vol. 45 (1970), pp. 493-496.

39. J. P. Geyman, "Family Practice in Evolution," *New England Journal of Medicine*, Vol. 298, No. 11 (Mar. 16, 1978), p. 596.

40. "Medical Education in the United States, 1979-1980," p. 2830, Table 4.

41. E. Charney, "Internal Medicine and Pediatric Education For Primary Care," *Journal of Medical Education* 130 (suppl.), December 1975.

42. J. P. Geyman, "Future Medical Priorities in the United States," *Journal of the American Medical Association*, Vol. 245, No. 11 (Mar. 20, 1981), p. 1140.

43. H. Wechsler, J. L. Dorsey, and J. D. Boney, "A Follow-up Study of Residents in Internal Medicine, Pediatrics and Obstetrics-Gynecology Training Programs in Massachusetts: Implications for Primary Care Physicians," *New England Journal of Medicine*, Vol. 298 (1978), pp. 15-21.

44. L. H. Aiken, C. E. Lewis, J. Craig et al., "The Contributions of Specialists to the Delivery of Primary Care: A New Perspective," *New England Journal of Medicine*, Vol. 300, No. 24 (June 14, 1979), pp. 1363-1370.

45. J. P. Geyman, "How Effective is the 'Hidden System' of Primary Care?" *Journal of Family Practice*, Vol. 9 (1979), pp. 563-564. M. L. Peterson, "The Place of the General Internist in Primary Care," *Annals of Internal Medicine*, Vol. 91 (1979), p. 305.

46. Institute of Medicine, *Aging and Medical Education*. (Washington, D.C.: National Academy of Sciences, 1978).

47. N. J. Cotsonas, H. G. Getz, and J. I. Newman in A. D. Hunt and L. E. Weeks (eds), *Medical Education since 1960*. (Lansing: Michigan State University Foundation, 1980), p. 61.

48. C. H. Bazuin and A. M. Yonke, "Improvement of Teaching Skills in a Clinical Setting," *Journal of Medical Education*, Vol. 53 (May 1978), p. 378.

49. J. W. Jones and P. O. Ways, in Hunt and Weeks, *op. cit.*, p. 154.

50. G. E. Miller, *Educating Medical Teachers*. (Cambridge: Harvard University Press, 1980), pp. 207-208.

51. D. Reisman, *Constraint and Variety in American Education*. (Garden City: Doubleday, 1958).

52. *Statistical Abstract of the United States*, 100th ed. (Washington: U.S. Department of Commerce, 1979), p. 116, Chart 180.

53. C. G. Sheps, "Education for What? A Decalogue for Change," *Journal of the American Medical Association*, Vol. 38, No. 3 (July 18, 1977), p. 234.

54. D. W. Seldin, "The Medical Model: Biomedical Science as the Basis of Medicine," in *Beyond Tomorrow*. (New York: Rockefeller University Press, 1977), pp. 38.

Chapter 5

Financing and Expenditures of the Academic Medical Center

GROWING CONCERN OVER FINANCE

A universal preoccupation of academic medical centers is the complicated issue of their financial health and stability. Addressing common purposes of education, research, patient care, and community services, modern academic medical centers often find that the final common denominator is money. Although activity and argument may be devoted to missions, goals, or objectives, the problem of choice usually focuses on the allocation of scarce budgetary resources or the development of new sources of revenue.

Until recently, the academic medical centers have been largely shielded from the need to make choices. A long postwar history of unparalleled financial riches and institutional expansion led deans, medical educators, researchers, physicians, and hospital administrators to expect a continuously enlarged cornucopia of funds, particularly from external sources, raised from the general public through government taxation or health insurance premiums.

But as the "days of wine and roses" began to draw to a close in the late 1960s, academic medical centers found themselves competing for funds with other institutional sectors of an increasingly specialized and fragmented society. Like these other sectors, academic medicine saw its character change in two significant respects. First, concern with financial issues became dominant. If politics is, in the terms of Harold Lasswell, the eminent political scientist, "who gets what, when and how," the "what" has very simply become money. Whether the politics are internal to the university world or external at the local, state, or federal level, the fierce competition for funds produces conflict and acrimony. Budgeting and finance are often said to be processes for the equitable distribution of dissatisfaction.

Second, to assure its ability to compete for funds, to be financially healthy, and to handle acrimony, the academic medical center has had to develop and recruit a new breed of financial managers. The strength of the financial management organization is increasingly evident in the decisionmaking process. The financial managers of academic medical centers exercise enormous power and influence, just as they do in all large-scale, multipurpose enterprises. This is especially true in the complex hospital financial and regulatory area, and it is increasingly so in the medical schools.

The growing power of the financial managers reflects not only their individual talents but also their expert knowledge of the intricacies of the external legislative, budgetary, regulatory, insurance, and administrative requirements to which the academic medical centers must conform in order to maintain financial stability. They thus exemplify the adage that knowledge is power. This knowledge extends far beyond simple understanding of accounting and budgeting principles or methods. It embraces the skillful manipulation of a segmented and uncoordinated system of grants, appropriations, fees for service, loans, and reimbursement or payment practices, and the shifting of medical center activities among the many sources of revenue so as to maximize the total resources available to the center without, presumably, sacrificing critical program goals or principles. Extensive commitments, such as faculty tenure, have been made under what now clearly appears to be "soft money:" thus the financial manager's expertness is in great demand.

These new developments—the frenetic concern with financial questions and the strength of the financial administrators—have serious implications for the institutional ethos of the academic medical center. The inherent conservatism of the financial administrator inevitably reinforces the naturally conservative bent of the faculty to resist programmatic change and alteration of traditional priorities. Faculty and departmental chairmen, sensing the decline in well-known sources of funds, are actively exploiting new opportunities to support what they regard as essential needs, current or prospective.

Academic medical centers admittedly are confronted with a serious predicament. As we shall see, their financial health is only partly in their own hands. They are attractive objects of philanthropic giving, and faculty seek out such sources aggressively. But inasmuch as resources of the medical school and the hospital are increasingly interchangeable, if not actually commingled, the financial health of the centers now depends less on tuition, research, and philanthropy and more upon funding for patient care. The overwhelming significance of the Medicare and Medicaid programs to the federal budget has shifted power over health affairs to those committees whose principal interest is in fiscal affairs, namely the Senate Finance Committee and the House Ways and Means Committee.

Like the newly powerful financial administrators of the academic medical centers, the members of these committees are also conservative in approach. They are more interested in controlling health costs than in improving health care organization or achieving equitable access to care. Thus, as the old health leadership sparked by Senator Lister Hill and Congressman John Fogarty has disappeared, and the recent federal programs of manpower and education support draw to a close, research levels are stabilized, at best, while the patient care and community service activity, managed principally under hospital leadership, emerges as the financial core of the academic medical center.

In reviewing the financial aspects of the academic medical center, we wish only to set forth the major components of the financial framework and their interaction. Many issues, such as the question of overhead allocations, will be deliberately left aside. We are well aware that the overhead issue burns fiercely in the breasts of all academic administrators, but the level of overhead is in part a question of total federal expenditures, in part a question of federal support of the alleged total cost of federally sponsored medical center activities, and finally a federal question of support of general higher education. The examination of these questions would take us far afield from our major concern.

Our objective is to delineate the relationship between the public interest and the academic medical centers as they adjust to new budgetary conditions (the decline in federal support for medical education and research and the new emphasis on control of health care costs). This chapter first outlines the overall budgetary dimensions of academic medical centers as a significant component of national health expenditures. Then we show the similarities and differences, among sources of financing, outline the implications thereof, and point to financing trends, especially in the public sector. Finally, to illustrate the conflicts, trends, and tensions within the centers as well as to sharpen our attention to public policy, we discuss at length public policies on financing of graduate medical education.

THE ACADEMIC MEDICAL CENTER IS "BIG BUSINESS"

As the academic medical centers evolved into their present central role in the American health care system, they came to account for a very substantial portion of our national health expenditures. Collectively and individually, they are in every sense "big business." In 1979 the medical schools and their 995 affiliated hospitals spent about $43 billion—$5 billion in the medical schools and $38 billion in the hospitals.[1] The $43 billion was 20 percent of our national health expenditures ($212 billion).[2]

More significantly, the expenditure of $38 billion for the affiliated hospitals was 45 percent of all national hospital expenditures ($85 billion). Of these 995 hospitals, 203 are federal, psychiatric, or long-term-care institutions. The remaining 792 are community hospitals, which spent $31 billion, or 45 percent of the total $66 billion spent by all 5842 community hospitals in the country. The largest and most costly of the community hospitals are the 325 or so members of the Council of Teaching Hospitals of the Association of American Medical Colleges. It is estimated that these COTH hospitals spent about $18.5 billion in 1979.[3] Thus, although these 325 major teaching hospitals are fewer than 6 percent of the nation's community hospitals, they account for 28 percent of the total community hospital expenditures—a meaningful attestation to their size, number of beds, and centrality in the health care system.

Although each academic center is a multimillion dollar business, their operating costs vary widely. Medical school budgets in 1979 ranged from $7.4 million to $116.3 million, with a median value of $39.5 million. Similarly, the major teaching community hospitals had an average annual budget in 1977 of about $45 million, ranging from a minimum of $4 million to a maximum of $219 million.[4] As shown in Table 1 the medical school and major teaching hospital are major financial ventures that together can well exceed a quarter of a billion dollars in operating costs.

Each of these centers has, of course, a number of additional major as well as limited hospital affiliations. Several medical schools in these centers are also part of a larger health education complex in their universities. If the costs of these other hospitals and schools were included, the total costs of each academic medical center would be vastly

Table 1.   Expenditures of Selected Academic Medical Centers, 1977-1978
(thousands of dollars)

	School	Hospital	Total
Albert Einstein/Montefiore[a]	$ 92,130	$173,325	$265,455
Columbia/Presbyterian[a]	112,778	151,050	263,828
Johns Hopkins University	83,370	88,282	171,652
University of Chicago	66,530	68,661	135,191
Duke University	67,360	65,747	133,107
Southwestern Medical School (Dallas)	70,330	47,774	118,104
University of Florida	33,320	28,424	61,744

Source: Association of American Medical Colleges, Liaison Committee for Medical
Education, "Annual Questionnaire," 1977-1978, 1978-1979; American Hospital Association, *Hospital Guide,* 1979 and 1980 editions.
[a]Data for these centers are for 1978-1979.

increased.

The university-owned hospital has been particularly attractive to
medical schools because such an arrangement makes possible a substantial measure of direct program control. There are now sixty-five
university-owned hospitals, of which forty-two are in state universities.
Apart from the state subsidies for the state-owned hospitals, university-
owned hospitals resemble other community teaching hospitals in their
financing and operations. Many university-owned hospitals have annual budgets of more than $100 million.[5] Like other institutions,
university-owned hospitals have found their costs rising markedly in
recent years, creating serious financial problems for their universities.
Many are now asking whether it is wise to continue such ownership
in view of competing demands for funds from other academic entities
and programs.

THE FINANCES OF MEDICAL SCHOOLS

The fiscal characteristics of medical schools and their affiliated
teaching hospitals are markedly dissimilar except in two major respects.
First, each institution is heavily dependent upon multiple sources of
revenue, most of them public sources—federal, state, and local government. Second, each has experienced a spectacular and steady budgetary
expansion. In the twenty years from 1959 to 1979 total reported medical
school expenditures increased from $319 million to $4.8 billion.[6] In the
same period, as the costs of hospital care in the nation rose from $9
billion to $85 billion,[7] the share of hospital expenditures attributable

to teaching hospitals increased sharply. For example, from 1973 to 1977 the costs of the COTH member hospitals increased from 20.8 percent to 27.9 percent of national hospital costs.[8]

But the differences in the financial characteristics of medical schools and teaching hospitals are more profound than their similarities. The first and most important difference relates to sources of revenue. Over 40 percent of medical school revenue is derived from public and private grants and contracts which are specifically restricted by the sponsor to targeted purposes, programs, or departments. Such funds are generally obtained through a spirited "entrepreneurial" activity on the part of faculty, notably in research.

In contrast, hospital revenues come overwhelmingly from third-party public and private payers or state subsidies for patient care. Like medical schools, hospitals also secure restricted lump sum revenues, and third-party payers, of course, restrict their payments for services rendered to their own eligibles. But the fundamental characteristic of hospital finance is that it is related to the single function of patient care, and revenues tend to be directly tied to the volume and scope of care, i.e., the costs or charges for individual patient services, either in inpatient wards or in outpatient clincis or emergency rooms.

As a consequence of these differences, medical school expenditures are for many different projects in research, education, or patient care, as shown in Table 2, whereas hospital expenditures tend to be mainly for patient care. Thus medical school financing exacerbates the inherent fragmentation of institutional purpose and objective, while teaching hospital financing supports the unitary objective of patient care.

Table 2.   Comparison of Medical School Expenditures, 1958–1959 and 1978–1979

	1958-1959	*1978-1979*
Number of Schools	85	125 [a]
Total expenditures (millions of dollars)	319.0	4,819.9
General operations	174.8	2,741.8
Sponsored/restricted	144.2	2,078.1
Research	113.7	1,099.3
Federal	74.1	882.6
Teaching and training	25.4	438.4
Federal	20.8	217.9
Health and community service	5.1	540.4

Source: "Medical Education in the United States 1979-1980," *Journal of the American Medical Association,* Vol. 244, No. 25, p. 2819 (Dec. 26, 1980), Table 24.
[a]Dollar figures are for 112 fully accredited schools.

A second significant difference is that, although both institutions are heavily dependent upon public funding, they look to different, even competing, parts of the public treasury. All hospitals depend heavily and increasingly upon Medicare and Medicaid funds. For example, in 1979 government paid for 56 percent of all hospital expenditures, but Medicare and Medicaid (both federal and state payments) alone constituted almost two-thirds of this revenue.[9] By contrast, medical schools depend principally on federal funds from the National Institutes of Health, the National Science Foundation, and the Bureau of Health Manpower. Federal funds as a proportion of total medical school revenues reached a peak of 54 percent in 1966, declining to 32 percent in 1977 and to 29 percent in 1979, although the absolute amount of federal funds continued to increase, from $481 million in 1966 to $1249 million in 1977 and $1433 million in 1979.[10] Schools and hospitals have competed for state appropriations, in some cases to support their general operations and in others to cover deficits in patient care operations, or to support specific programs of education and research.

Most medical schools are not isolated or independent organizations. Rather, the medical school is often an integral part of a larger academic complex, and it is not always possible to distinguish medical school revenues and expenditures with complete accuracy. A hospital, on the other hand, is a separate organizational entity whose total costs are not difficult to ascertain and even to control, although it may be difficult to estimate the cost of its different functions.

The financial arrangements between medical schools and hospitals, both affiliated and university-owned, are very intricate, often informal, and not at all standard. Each academic medical center has its own arrangements or rules for the generation and disposition of revenue or accounting for expenditures. Most importantly, arrangements are frequently established at a departmental level. Ad hoc arrangements of mutual convenience abound, as does conflict over the division of revenues or the responsibility for costs--particularly when both institutions are supporting the same type of activities. For example, although residents and interns are usually paid by hospitals from patient care revenues, many programs to train family practice residents are also financed by grants to or contracts with medical schools. Usually, as described in Chapter 4, medical schools also tend to secure the funds for subspecialty fellowship training, even though the fellows work in the hospital and perform patient-care functions.

Clinical faculty are largely but not exclusively financed on medical school budgets. In many cases, affiliated or university-owned hospitals pay the salaries of full-time clinical academic faculty who are substantially engaged in research and teaching as well as patient-care responsibilities. Therefore, the issues surrounding payment for clinical services of teaching physicians involve issues of institutional policy, engendering deep-seated conflicts within the center about the distribution of revenue between school and hospital, the remuneration of faculty members, and the relevant academic criteria for promotion of clinical faculty. In addition, of course, there is the long-standing and unsettled controversy about possible "double-billing" by teaching physicians under Part A (hospital services) and Part B (physicians' services) under Medicare.

Although medical schools are supported by multiple sources of revenue, they are not all of equal significance, as shown in Table 3. Several observations seem significant:

1. General operating funds are derived from many sources, while sponsored and restricted funds are largely federal grants and contracts. State and local government and nongovernment grants and contracts are far less frequent than the federal commitment.
2. Funds from state and local governments are provided basically as general operating revenue, whereas federal general operating funds are available only for overhead or indirect costs. These nonfederal public funds are mainly for the 66 public schools.
3. Professional fees and hospital and clinics are a major revenue source, a substantial amount of which is internally restricted for eventual use.
4. Tuition and philanthropy, once the major source of medical school revenue, are now relatively unimportant.

Most of the revenue is expended on programs of instruction and research, as seen in Table 4, but significant costs are also incurred for various support functions, such as administrative overhead, libraries, computer centers, and plant operation and maintenance. In some instances, other units may directly support medical school activities and requirements, but the funds may not be recorded in medical school accounts. Almost 25 percent of general operating expenditures is so classified.

Similar information on revenue and expenditures has not been assembled in studies for all the affiliated hospitals of academic medical centers. But university-owned hospitals substantially resemble other community hospitals in their pattern of payment or reimbursement for patient care, with private and public third-party payers for patient care being the predominant sources of funds. A recent survey by the Council of Teaching Hospitals of the income of university-owned hospitals is summarized in Table 5. The overwhelming dependence upon

Table 3. Operating Revenues of U. S. Medical Schools, 1976–1977 through 1978–1979

Item	1976-1977		1977-1978		1978-1979		Range, Thousands of $s		
	No. of Schools	Amount, Millions of $	No. of Schools	Amount, Millions of $	No. of Schools	Amount, Millions of $	Min.	Median	Max.
Total Revenues	112	3,940	112	4,316	112	4,906	7,534	39,463	116,293
General operating	112	2,197	112	2,451	112	2,623	3,702	23,947	71,290
State and local government	101	805	100	899	98	1,023	9	9,739	38,469
Appropriations to public schools	65	729	86	822	66	944	2,879	12,953	38,489
Subsidies	35	76	34	77	32	80	9	1,803	12,693
Professional fee income (medical service plan)	78	440	75	481	73	558	88	6,340	24,247
Recovery of indirect costs on grants and contracts	108	241	94	237	91	269	3	1,806	15,338
Federal	106	223	92	215	90	244	3	1,568	13,101
Nonfederal	73	18	86	22	83	25	3	170	2,235
Tuition and fees	112	194	112	231	112	265	67	2,006	10,232
Endowment income (unrestricted)	53	48	51	53	52	56	2	342	7,844
Gifts (unrestricted)	70	36	65	50	68	61	1	322	15,441
Income from college services	65	37	62	42	62	52	1	328	8,413
General university funds	38	85	37	85	38	96	23	2,397	9,882

(Cont. on next page)

Table 3 (Continued)

Item	1976-1977		1977-1978		1978-1979		Range, Thousands of $s		
	No. of Schools	Amount, Millions of $	No. of Schools	Amount, Millions of $	No. of Schools	Amount, Millions of $	Min.	Median	Max.
Hospitals and clinics	45	215	43	226	48	231	6	2,420	12,991
Miscellaneous sources	89	96	72	148	76	163	1	333	22,448
Sponsored and restricted programs	112	1,743	112	1,865	112	2,078	43	13,058	87,010
Grants and contracts									
Federal	112	1,047	112	1,079	112	1,189	43	7,233	42,382
State and local	93	206	95	214	100	232	5	655	26,931
Nongovernment	110	279	110	322	110	346	41	2,293	13,753
Income used for administratively restricted programs	58	213	61	250	61	311	1	1,768	28,723
Professional fee income	31	113	33	135	32	171	226	2,240	22,523
Hospitals and clinics	16	53	15	59	18	74	12	3,168	16,295
State funds	17	20	14	24	13	26	33	802	9,293
Other	32	27	35	32	34	40	1	367	18,393

Source: "Medical Education in the United States, 1979–1980," *Journal of the American Medical Association*, Vol. 244, No. 25, p. 2820 (Dec. 26, 1980), Table 25.

Table 4. U. S. Medical School Expenditures by Function, 1978–1979 (millions of dollars)

Function	Grand Total	General Operating			Sponsored and Restricted Programs
		Total	Recorded in Medical School Accounts	Not Recorded in Medical School Accounts	
Total expenditures	$4,820	$2,742	$2,093	$649	$2,078
Instruction and departmental research	1,794	1,356	1,247	109	438
Research	1,184	85	37	48	1,099
Health services	687	366	157	209	320
Multipurpose	177	63	27	36	114
Academic support	249	201	175	26	48
Institutional support	293	283	183	100	10
Operation and maintenance of physical plant	264	260	189	72	4
Student services	39	36	29	7	3
Scholarships and fellowships	50	23	14	9	27
Other	83	68	36	32	14

Source: "Medical Education in the United States, 1979–1980," *Journal of the American Medical Association,* Vol. 244, No. 25, p. 2821 (Dec. 26, 1980), Table 26.

Table 5. Sources of Income in University-owned Hospitals, Fiscal Year 1977

Source	Public (N=42) Amount ($000)	% of Total	Private (N=20) Amount ($000)	% of Total	Total (N=62) Amount ($000)	% of Total
Medicare	389,037	19.6	344,555	27.1	733,592	22.5
Blue Cross	273,751	13.8	296,340	23.3	570,091	17.5
Commercial insurance	361,485	18.2	205,629	16.2	567,114	17.4
Medicaid	305,772	15.4	186,267	14.7	492,039	15.1
State appropriations	311,863	15.7	30,788	2.4	342,651	10.5
Additional government payments	68,430	3.5	14,524	1.1	82,954	4.6
Self-pay	145,582	7.3	136,825	10.8	282,407	8.7
Other	128,719	6.5	56,573	4.4	185,292	5.7
Total	1,984,639	100.0	1,271,537	100.0	3,256,176	100.0

Source: Council of Teaching Hospitals, Association of American Medical Colleges, *Toward a More Contemporary Public Understanding of the Teaching Hospital* (Washington, D.C., 1979), Table 12, (p. 51).

Medicare/Medicaid, insurance, and other public funds at both private and state-owned hospitals is immediately evident. Payments from these third-party sources totaled 86 percent of all revenues.

NEW REVENUE SOURCES AND
NEW PROBLEMS

Because their sources of revenue are so different, trends in medical school and hospital financing have to be separately examined. Since the late 1960s the changes in financing of medical schools have been very dramatic. General operating revenues have risen from 42 percent of total revenues in 1969 to 58 percent in 1979.[11] This shift to general operating revenues has been more pronounced in the public schools, reflecting their ability to turn to state government as an alternative funding source as the federal funding for research, education, and service demonstration grants and contracts has leveled off or ended. In 1978-1979, for example, 65.3 percent of the funding for public schools was received as general operating revenues, compared to only 48.3 percent in the private schools.

The decline in restricted revenues has occurred especially in federal funding for research which fell (from 29 percent of the total in 1969 to 18 percent in 1979) and for teaching and training (down from 12 percent to 4.4 percent). These are relative, not absolute, declines in funds. To pay for expanded operations, to establish new medical schools, and to compensate for general inflation, both general and restricted revenues, including federal funds, have grown in current dollar terms, as shown in the previous tables. The growth in real terms, however, has been substantially less. For example, for a cohort of 91 schools, restricted revenues rose over $1 billion from 1970 to 1979, at a compound average annual rate of 10 percent but in real terms, the increase in funding was only 3.1 percent. At the same time, general revenues have shown larger increases. For the same 91 schools, general revenues increased over $1.6 billion, or 15.5 percent per year compounded in current dollars and about 5 percent in real terms.[12] At least in theory, the movement from restricted to general revenues should have provided school administrators more flexibility to adjust to changing times.

Overall, during the 1970s, funds for all medical schools rose about 13.4 percent a year in current dollars, an increase in real terms of 6.5 percent a year compounded. According to the Association of American Medical Colleges, this increase has been roughly equal to the increase in the number of students taught by medical school faculties. The implication is misleading, however, since the education of undergraduate medical students constitutes only a small fraction of faculty activities.

The problems of financing have compelled medical schools to examine the sources of their revenue. As shown earlier, tuition fees and endowments or philanthropy are only a small part of school income. Even with the very substantial annual increases that have lifted tuitions to over $10,000 in some schools, tuition and fees still constitute only 5-6 percent of total medical school revenues. Even in private schools, where there are only small state subsidies, tuition and fees account for only 8.5 percent of total revenue. Endowment income actually declined from 2.1 percent to 1.1 percent of total medical school revenue during the 1970s, the drop naturally being more severe in private schools.

Over the long term the financial health of medical schools seems to have become dependent in both absolute and relative terms on funds from two sources. These are the increased support provided by state governments to private as well as to public medical schools, and the production of large-scale revenue through professional practice fees or other income under faculty medical service plans and in hospitals and clinics.

State appropriations to public schools in the 1970s increased from $170 million, or 12 percent of total medical school revenues, to $944 million, or 19 percent of total revenues. These increases reflect two broad considerations. First, most of the medical schools founded after World War II were state schools. Many did not move into full-scale operation until the 1970s. Second, as public schools, they were expected to be responsive to public pressures, supported by the incentive of public appropriations, for primary care, family practice, better distribution of physicians, or increased total health manpower. In addition, apart from a limited amount of state grants for restricted programs, state governments began to provide a new subsidy of private schools, often in the form of capitation grants tied to the number of in-state students admitted. The amount of state funds for these purposes rose from $18 million (1.3 percent of total school revenue) in 1968-1969 to $80 million (1.6 percent of total school revenue) in 1978-1979. (See Table 3.)

Chapter 3 broadly outlined some of the implications of the drive in medical schools to develop income via more extensive medical practice, especially on the fee-for-service basis. This subject was of sufficient concern that in 1977 the Association of American Medical Colleges completed a comprehensive two-year study of medical practice plans. It has also recently published the results of its 1980 survey of this feature of medical school organization and financing.[13]

Patient-care activities have, of course, traditionally been viewed as one of the primary activities of clinical faculty members. Until recently, however, practice income was a minor source of revenue. After World War II, faculty were normally employed on a fixed compensation basis, with revenue derived from grants, contracts, or other regular sources. Fees for clinical care were usually retained by the school or the university.

In time, the term *medical practice plan* developed to identify any regular system for managing the financial and other aspects of medical practice for the full-time clinical faculty. "Volunteer" or "part-time" clinical faculty, e.g., community physicians, are not covered by such plans, their clinical practices being regarded as outside the purview of the university control mechanisms.

As financial access to medical care has expanded enormously over the past twenty-five years, more extensive income opportunities have become available to support the academic medical center. Especially with Medicare and Medicaid, care that had earlier been provided "free" became a major potential source of income for the academic medical center. Thus, practice plans have come into being for governance of medical practice arrangements and for distribution of income among the institutions—departments and top management—and the faculty, clinical and nonclinical.

Not all schools have organized practice plans, but they are growing rapidly. In 1980, eighty-seven faculty practice plans were reported to be in operation, up almost 30 percent from 1977, when there were sixty-seven such plans. Professional fee income from faculty practice plans increased from $90 million in 1970 (5.8 percent of total reported medical school revenues) to $727 million in 1978-1979 (14.8 percent of total school revenues.)

Professional fee income can be used very flexibly by the academic medical center. Thus, it is of importance that the $727 million reported by just 87 schools is almost 26 percent of the total general operating revenue of *all* schools. For the school that reported the greatest total revenues ($116.3 million) in 1978-1979, professional fee income was almost $45 million, or 40 percent of the total. For the median school such income amounted to 22 percent of the total reported income.

In addition to the income from faculty practice plans, medical schools realized $355 million in 1978-1979 from the operation of hospitals and clinics, amounting to 7.2 percent of total school revenues. Thus, in that year income from the delivery of health services from fees and hospitals provided 22.2 percent of the grand total of $4.9 billion of school revenues.

In parallel with the trend to increase income from patient care services there has been a move to put full-time faculty (not just the traditional hospital-based physicians in radiology, pathology, and anaesthesiology) on hospital payrolls. Although this practice is widespread, its financial dimensions are uncertain. Obviously, whether salaries are met by fee income or hospital operating budgets, there are academic questions of faculty status and program issues of the nature of the patient care effort. But the budgeting and fiscal issues are of rather special concern and produce persistent internal tensions. In general terms, the issues concern the division of resources between the hospital and the medical school as institutions. They thus raise directly questions of program emphasis and the relative power of the dean, hospital director, and department heads. More specifically, the maintenance and continued increase of the personal income of the clinical faculty is a very serious point in controversy, going to the very heart of the full-time faculty concept. To the extent that these income issues are resolved by increasing personal income of individual clinical faculty to levels approximating those of physicians in private practice, the effect is to obscure and neglect departmental, school, or hospital purposes that may be served by use of such income. From the school's perspective for example, the more fee income available to the department chairmen or dean, the more potential support for research, teaching, and school overhead. Conversely, the more income distributed to or retained by the hospital director, the more resources available for patient-care support, including the extension of health services not now provided, or the improvement of existing systems of health services.

These questions are very complicated in a large, multiinstitutional academic medical center, whether one focuses on income from faculty practice plans or on the inclusion of revenue from hospital or clinics in the medical school budget, or on expenditures for full-time staff directly on the hospital budget. The issues go to the heart of the "joint product" approach which we have earlier discussed. Health services revenues are not usually allocated with a view to where the logic of program plans and missions would move the hospital or medical school as a total institution. Rather, the power of the medical school, especially the department chairmen, tends to predominate, and the departmental needs are often regarded as primary. Thus, in negotiations among school and hospital officials and clinical faculty, the income distribution decisions tend to reflect less the logic of the institutional situation and more the power and prestige of departmental chairmen. If there is any prospect that the hospital can finance the teaching faculty out of its more flexible reimbursement sources, medical school pressure tends to assure that such action will be taken. It is of no minor import that in 1979 over 52 percent of all full-time hospital physicians, excluding house staff, in all U.S. hospitals were in COTH hospitals, whereas in 1973 the proportion was only 42.5 percent. [14]

This trend to support faculty from health services income has been fraught with dangerous conflicts and equally dangerous portents for the future. How much practice income should be returned to the clinical faculty who generate the income has become a major issue not only within the school but also between the teaching hospital and the school. In the years during which the academic medical center was developing into its present form, voluntary or part-time clinical faculty were increasingly replaced by faculty on full-time academic status, who received a regular salary with only a minor dependence, if any, upon practice income. The incentives created by high private-practice incomes have already partially eroded this system. As government moves away from regulation, direction, and financial support toward a policy of encouraging competition among health care provider organizations, these conflicts will become more serious and frequent.

But the conflict over health services income distribution has programmatic features as well. The range of conflict between the teaching hospital and the school has been enlarged. As a consequence of the stress on provider marketing, the teaching hospital, already faced with a decline in patient referrals, especially for tertiary care, must take the lead to seek out new and, if possible, defined populations to serve. Rare is the medical school, given the historical stress on research and specialty training and indifference or even hostility to large-scale health services, that can readily conform to such a hospital strategy. Clashes will be inevitable when the hospital goes in a direction that various units in the medical school oppose. Disagreement will be especially sharp because the hospital may well have to compete with other community hospitals that are less saddled with major educational costs—the obvious costs of house staff stipends, the less obvious costs of teaching medical students, and the still less obvious costs of supervision of house staff and the various indirect educational costs of the hospital, all of which are largely covered by patient care revenues.

Within the academic medical center, then, the finances of the school and its affiliated teaching hospitals require joint examination. This is rarely, if ever, done. The heart of the relationship is in the concept of joint production. Individual medical school faculty, according to Association of American-Medical Colleges surveys, have from one to four areas of responsibility (teaching, research, patient care, and administration). As shown in Table 6, only a small percentage report a single area of responsibility. About 80 percent of the faculty report responsibilities for patient care, usually in combination with teaching, research, and/or administration.

Table 6. Areas of Responsibility of Full-Time Medical School Faculty, 1977–1978

	M.D. Degree		Ph.D. Degree	
Areas of Responsibility	*Number*	*Percent*	*Number*	*Percent*
One area of responsibility				
Teaching	1,034	4.0	315	2.8
Research	396	1.5	1,262	11.3
Patient care	537	2.0	34	0.3
Administration	247	0.9	87	0.8
Other	31	0.1	20	0.2
Two areas of responsibility				
Teaching and research	1,878	7.2	6,013	54.0
Teaching and patient care	4,322	16.5	226	2.0
Teaching and administration	437	1.7	137	1.2
Other combination of two	309	1.2	238	2.1
Three areas of responsibility				
Teaching, research, and patient care	7,896	30.1	752	6.8
Teaching, research, and administration	824	3.1	1,095	9.8
Teaching, patient care, and administration	1,830	7.0	84	0.8
Other combination of three	266	1.0	167	1.5
Four areas of responsibility				
Teaching, research, patient care, and administration	4,976	19.0	410	3.7
Other combination of four	163	0.6	63	0.6
All other combinations	233	0.9	31	0.3
Subtotal	25,379	96.8	10,934	98.2
Unknown responsibilities	830	3.2	201	1.8
Total	26,209	100.0	11,135	100.0

Source: Association of American Medical Colleges, *Medical Education: Institutions, Characteristics and Programs.* (Washington, D.C.: AAMC, 1979), Figure 15, p. 16.

THE FINANCES OF TEACHING HOSPITALS

Several special features of the finances of teaching hospitals now require consideration. Even though these hospitals differ in size, ownership, goals, community service, research, and internal organization, they all share some level of commitment to clinical medical education. Consequently, they tend to incur higher costs than nonteaching hospitals of similar size when measured by almost any commonly used yardstick—total cost, per diem cost, cost per admission, or cost per case for a particular diagnosis.

It is difficult to identify all the sources of teaching hospitals' higher costs. In addition to direct educational costs, such as stipends and faculty teaching, several other factors raise costs: the need for tertiary-care facilities essential to the modern teaching hospital, the referral of sicker patients from outlying areas, and the intensity of service i.e., the high utilization of ancillary services related to these two service factors, as well as to the needs of students and house staff to learn by doing. Because of the great diversity in hospitals (in terms of the size and types of house staff and full-time staff, the extent and strength of the medical school affiliation, the character and size of outpatient services, diagnostic case mix, etc), definitive analyses of the higher costs of teaching hospitals have yet to be made. One fact is clear—the costs of hospitals of the academic medical centers continue to rise faster than the national average of 12-15 percent.[15] (See Table 7.) This long-term disproportionate increase in teaching hospital costs is of concern to both policymakers and medical center administrators because the issue of health cost containment has become so central to health policy.

Although the hospitals of the academic medical centers, including the university-owned hospitals, resemble other institutions in their dependence upon third-party patient care payments, certain special payment trends appear to be developing in teaching hospitals. Whereas the medical schools, even the private ones, are relying increasingly on general state appropriations, the reverse is true in the teaching hospitals. University-owned hospitals, for example, receive such funds primarily as subsidies for their clinical teaching and other educational activity and as an additional source of revenue for the care of medical-

Table 7. Costs of Nonfederal, Short-term Hospitals, 1973–1977

	1973	1975	1976	1977	*Increase 1973–1977*
Cost per Admission					
COTH members	$1293	$1888	$1897	$2383	84%
All U. S. hospitals	994	1165	1324	1509	52%
Cost per Day					
COTH members	139	209	236	271	95%
All U. S. Hospitals	128	151	173	198	55%

Source: Council of Teaching Hospitals, Association of American Medical Colleges, *Toward a More Contemporary Public Understanding of the Teaching Hospital* (Washington, D.C., 1979), Table 6, (p. 44).

ly indigent patients. Recently there has been a steady decline in the percentage contribution of state appropriations to university-owned teaching hospitals—from a high of 28 percent in 1970 to a low of 17 percent in 1977. (In absolute terms, state contributions increased over these years.)

While the relative importance of state funds declined, the role of Medicare funds in the hospital budget increased. Medicare's share of revenue of hospitals receiving state general appropriations rose from 11.4 percent in 1971 to 20.2 percent in 1977. In the private university-owned hospitals, which do not receive state appropriations, Medicare's share is, of course, even higher, reaching 26 percent in 1977. Blue Cross, commercial insurance, and Medicaid are the other major payers in the teaching hospitals, covering 45-55 percent of hospital revenue, depending upon a variety of factors, including availability of state appropriations.[16]

Despite current federal budget policy to slow the rise in Medicare expenditures and to reduce payments to hospitals, the dominant role of Medicare in the nation's hospital finances will become even stronger in the next fifteen years. In 1979, Medicare paid 25.4 percent of all hospital bills in the nation. In 1970, it paid less than 18 percent.[17] The Social Security Administration has projected that by 1990 12.6 percent of the total population will be 65 or older and 5.4 percent over 75, compared with 9.7 percent and 3.8 percent respectively, in 1970. The federal government's share of national health expenditures is expected to rise several percentage points from its present level of about 29 percent, an increase caused primarily by the rise in Medicare benefit payments.[18]

In all hospitals, perhaps most of all in the teaching hospitals, care of the aged patient will markedly increase. At present, Medicare eligibles account for one-third of all inpatient days.[19] This proportion will surely increase or the Medicare program will be amended to provide for alternative methods of care.

Medicare's dominant role has both financial and programmatic implications which policymakers and academics alike must take into account. On the financial side, government policy on Medicare will set the pattern for all third-party payers on rules and coverages for hospital reimbursement, e.g., financing of medical education, medical malpractice, or the special needs of the teaching hospital. Just as the financing of medical schools was dominated by federal research funding (as other funding sources always recognized), so will the financing of the teaching hospital be dominated by one large payer, Medicare.

But financing, of course, has programmatic implications. We believe that financial control by Medicare can help lead the medical schools to confront the problems of "the graying of America." Medical schools cannot ignore this trend in financing the hospital care and health services upon which medical education programs depend. It is impossible first as a matter of public policy, and second for the institutional survival of the medical school. Succinctly stated, the public interest in this demographic change means that the academic medical center must both prepare the future physician and also ready itself for the task of caring for a growing geriatric population.

CONSEQUENCES OF CONSTRAINED FEDERAL FUNDING

Public policy respecting the financing of academic medical centers is surely changing, to a large extent for federal budgetary reasons deriving from overall national economic considerations but also in response to concerns about the substance of federal health policy. The Reagan administration has greatly accelerated the spending reductions initiated under President Carter, both in the social service and entitlement programs of welfare, social security, Medicare and Medicaid and in the health programs that supported the academic medical center more directly. At the same time that the level of research grants at medical schools is being stabilized, the federal government has eliminated capitation grants and greatly curtailed student loans and other assistance. Also, it is implicitly accepting and acting upon the forecasts of a physician surplus. In lieu of regulatory measures to limit hospital costs or revenues, a federal health policy appears to be emerging that will promote a competitive model that franchises consumers equally and, in effect, puts hospitals and doctors at risk in large competitive organizations. These policies would depart from past concepts of health care as a "right" and operate according to the concept that health care is an economic good in a retail market, where providers compete and consumers choose.[20] It is an open question whether the new policies will differentiate the academic medical centers among the providers.

It is not easy to assess the seriousness of the financial situation facing the academic medical center. Reasonably assured of a continued level of funding for research, medical schools will find that their primary traditional objectives are unchallenged. The elimination of capitation grants is not really serious because such funding has never been a major resource for most schools. At least in theory, schools are better able than hospitals to structure themselves to absorb reductions because their multipurpose character gives them flexibility to choose among certain education programs and certain research activities. In reality, however, medical schools tend to regard any cut in the support of any activity as a disaster. Hospitals have much less discretion in absorbing budgetary reductions. It is true that they can always find efficiencies in overhead or support services, and thus reduce costs. They could also diminish their use of technology. But by and large, if the hospital has fewer funds or must face stringent cost controls, it can only respond by reducing the volume, scope, or level of patient-care services.

Above all, the hospitals in the academic medical center are not independent or free agents. Like other hospitals, they must function within the framework of the entire reimbursement and delivery system, and as teaching hospitals, they must especially fit the ways that medical schools and faculty physicians behave.

PUBLIC POLICY AND THE SEARCH FOR FINANCIAL STABILITY

It is extremely difficult, and perhaps unwise, to attempt to separate financing issues of public policy in health from other, presumably substantive, issues of health policy. Given the systemic nature of health care problems, the examination of health policies may start from many vantage points (e.g., education, services, research, or manpower distribution). In general, however, all examinations tend to identify the same specific problems of access to care, quality of care, regionalization of services, etc. As we have stressed, actions to serve the public interest in access to quality health care at reasonable cost require changes and new policies at many interrelated points in the health system.

This fact was recognized by the Graduate Medical Education National Advisory Committee (GMENAC) in its studies and in its proposals to the Secretary of Health and Human Services which were discussed earlier. A major study conducted by the Urban Institute on behalf of GMENAC analyzed the interrelations among several financing policies for medical education: capitation grants to medical schools, size and deployment of the National Health Service Corps through award of scholarships, other student loans and scholarships, hospital cost controls and reimbursement, payments for services of teaching physicians, and modifications to Medicare/Medicaid regulations to group hospitals by size and teaching status.[21] The basic criteria by which the study evaluated policy options were encouragement of primary care services, especially to the underserved, equitable access of entry into the medical profession, and efficiency in education and overall health care cost control. The Institute found that the best route lay in changes in the reimbursement system, especially in physician fee structure, but it recognized that such changes could be made only as part of comprehensive health system reforms.

Over the years ahead a number of health financing issues will be widely discussed, with special relevance to the problems of academic medical centers. Can long-term financial stability be created for the academic medical center? How should the cost be distributed between the short-term beneficiaries (students) and the long-term beneficiary (society-at-large)? Is there a new, definable, and limited federal role to replace its multiple and broad-ranging activities of the past three decades? Will we make a major move to a health-care marketing and business model which gives greater weight to efficiency and less weight to equity achieved through regulation? Do teaching hospitals have special financial needs that cost control, competition, and planning policies ought to recognize? Should we allow technology to be introduced into the health care system on the basis of "provider risk" in a competitive framework, or should we insist that safety, effectiveness, and efficacy first be tested, evaluated, and approved (as in current Food and Drug Administration practice)? Is biomedical research and research training adequately funded to meet legitimate societal needs? Should the private sector, especially business and industry, be expected to enlarge its financial support of such research activities?

It is easier to inventory the financial problems confronting the academic medical centers than to prescribe the solutions. But an essential first step toward solutions is to recognize that the problems go far beyond those of inadequate total funding or highly restricted funding from one source. Although the centers all want more funds, it is perhaps critical, as we discuss later, that they lack a system of governance that creates a framework of choice among competing priorities.

The radical difficulty of the academic medical center is that it knows only one philosophy, namely that of continued expansion. But, paradoxically, in the current period of "no growth," part of the financing problem of centers is the attainment of financial stability. Can they achieve this stability and the assurance to undertake what they want when the overriding public policies are likely to be those of competition in the marketplace?

Each financing issue raises a different perspective for public policymakers—as well as for officials in academic medicine. For example, how to undergird and support medical education is a long-term question, but how to pay for the care of the individual patient in the hospital is more a short-term, immediate question. Genuine financial stability for the academic medical center is attainable only within a framework of regionalization and orderly planning, which is not easily reconciled with a philosophy of continued expansion under which each medical center attempts to attain a maximum size and to become a comprehensive education, research, and patient-care complex.

Stability in finance or in program has different meanings for the different segments of the academic medical center. Fondly recalling the growth years of 1950 to 1970, the researcher sees stability as meaning growth to expand upon past experiments or discoveries or to afford research opportunities to newly trained researchers. The hospital administrator, in contrast, is responsible for meeting the costs of a constantly more expensive "consumer product," that is, patient care. Perhaps that is why he approaches financing stability in terms of "purifying" patient care costs by moving responsibility for payment for graduate medical education to other funding sources.

AN EXAMPLE: GRADUATE MEDICAL EDUCATION

History teaches us that public policy is rarely totally overhauled. Rather, the traditional American political pattern is to modify selectively and incrementally. It is beyond our scope here to cover the entire field of medical center financing issues in detail. We are sure, however, that one of the unavoidable issues affecting the academic medical center is that of the cost and financing of graduate medical education. It is worth discussing at some length, in part because it will be at the forefront of policy debates and in part because it so well illustrates the complex external pressures upon the centers and points up the need for clear internal governance systems and procedures.

Graduate medical education (GME) has come under increasing scrutiny during the past five to ten years. It has been the subject of numerous studies and a spate of articles in the professional journals.[22] Two broad considerations have heightened this interest. First, as the costs of patient care have continued to mount relentlessly, third-party payers, public and private, have searched for ways to transfer costs apparently unrelated to patient care, such as those of GME, to other payers, to individual beneficiaries, or to education appropriations. Second, as we have seen in Chapter 4, there is a growing conviction that academic medicine has not been training the "right" kind of doctors. It has been suggested that government control the size of the pool of specialty manpower through laws that require increased efforts in primary-care graduate medical education and/or direct appropriations for the support of family medicine and primary care GME. Some of these proposals have been legislatively enacted.

If concern over costs and access to care have prompted public policy attention to GME, we need to be clear about certain aspects of the nature of graduate medical education. Two key considerations must be added to the analysis already presented in Chapter 4. In the first place, the pressures for service by teaching hospitals, the availability of foreign medical graduates, and the easy funding through third parties and the National Institutes of Health have distorted the purposes of residency training. As Rogers and Blendon note in their discussion of the causes of tension between government and the academic medical center, "it was primarily service needs, not education needs, that shaped the house staff training programs offered by academic medical centers.[23] The house staff met the enormous demands of hospital coverage, replacing those clinical faculty who preferred to concentrate on research, supporting those clinical specialists who maintained an interest in special and complex cases, and covering the needs for generalist care that the voluntary attending physicians did not provide in the outpatient clinics, the emergency room, or the inpatient wards.

The second point is that, despite these distortions, residency training became a broad learning experience constituting specialty education. Originally, the residency was simply vocational training—the young doctor's first full-time job experience, under the sole direction of the hospital. In time, residency training became part of the continuum of medical education by moving to sponsorship by the university and of its medical school. Eventually, medical schools assumed responsibility for over 90 percent of graduate medical education.

In the mid-1960s, two important reports provided the necessary blessing for this development. The Millis Commission on Graduate Medical Education, headed by Dr. John S. Millis, endorsed GME as a continuous program for the development of specialists, including physicians in primary care. It also recommended that university medical centers develop a corporate responsibility for residency training. This commission, a citizens' group sponsored by the American Medical Association, was paralleled by a special planning committee of the Association of American Medical Colleges, chaired by Dr. Lowell T. Coggeshall. The Coggeshall report, *Planning for Medical Progress through Education,* promoted even more strongly the proposition that the university should be the effective center of all aspects of medical education, and that the greatest possible effort should be made to move in the direction of university responsibility for graduate medical education.[24]

As the university took charge of graduate medical education during the 1960s, three other changes occurred. First, rotating internships were abolished. Second, more community hospitals sought medical school affiliations. And third, control of GME clearly came to rest with the training director, usually the department chairman in the medical school. Given his other powers over research proposals, grants and research training, clinical clerkships, and space and administrative support, the department chairman became the dominant executive in governance of both medical schools and hospitals.

The move to medical school responsibility raised a further question which lies at the heart of much of the substantive concern about the appropriate financing of graduate medical education. How can the academic medical center be held accountable for the number and types of specialists produced? When the decision to undergo residency training represented only an individual vocational choice to acquire specialist capabilities, and when the nation was not attempting to formulate an overall national health program, there was no question of matching numbers and types of residency positions to overall national manpower needs. Individual students went on to residency posts if their personal interests so dictated, otherwise, they went directly into practice after their internship. Today it is expected that all M.D. graduates will complete a residency before practice.

Yet as we approach a "doctor glut" in an era when medical practice has been totally changed, the total number of residency posts in the nation must match the number of medical school graduates. The content of the match, the number of specialists of each type, and the impact upon costs are in the forefront of discussions about financing GME. But what institutions will be designated to establish the match—specialty boards, medical schools, department chairmen, hospitals, the AMA? Or government?[25]

These are some of the significant unresolved considerations within the academic medical centers that are part of the framework for considering the cost and financing of graduate medical education. As to cost, the salaries or stipends of residents and fellows, along with fringe benefits, amounted to $1.4 billion in 1978-1979, less than 1 percent of national health expenditures.[26] But no valid estimates exist of such substantial additional costs as supervision, teaching, and the whole range of necessary educational support functions, not to mention the indirect hospital and medical school costs or the overutilization of hospital services generally endorsed by most medical educators as an unavoidable part of the learning process for students and residents.

Whatever the "true" cost of graduate medical education, determinations of the total amount and the allocations to beneficiaries are bound to be fairly arbitrary judgments, because graduate medical education is an integral part of the joint production process so characteristic of the academic medical center. Residents themselves provide direct patient care, assist other physicians to deliver patient care, learn from faculty and senior residents and in turn teach medical students in clerkships, and even occasionally engage in research. Studies show that residents spend about 70 percent of their time in patient care,[27] but this fact hardly solves the cost allocation problem. In the first place, the distribution of time varies by specialty. Moreover, "joint product" and "joint cost" considerations inevitably produce arbitrary judgments, derived from differing values, about the purpose as well as the cost of any activity, including patient care. And residents often participate in more than one activity at the same time.

The essence of the problem of paying for GME is typical of any joint product situation: any new program in the academic medical center must cover the incremental costs of the program itself plus some portion of "joint costs." Thus, if funding for any ongoing GME program is cut—or shifted—the cost of the remaining programs of the academic medical center must go up to assure that all joint costs are met. In contrast to the business world, there is no market by which costs can be transferred to one selling entity where cost recovery is relatively easy; thus the assignment of joint costs to differing payers or funds is bound to be arbitrary. This problem is not peculiar to graduate medical education, but illustrates the more general problems of disaggregating the costs of the academic medical center and of changing present methods of financing these costs.

These are the factors at work when we ask who now pays for GME, what is wrong with the present arrangements, and what options for change might be desirable. Patient-care revenues, largely from third-party payers, cover 70-80 percent of GME stipends. Over 50 percent of the cost is met by Medicare, Medicaid, the Veterans Administration, NIH, and other federal funding agencies.

Several arguments may be raised against this system of paying for GME predominantly through patient-care revenues:

1. Patients should not have to pay for education costs.
2. Accountability for numbers and types of residents rests largely with the medical school, but the funds are paid to the hospital.
3. With the coming physician surplus, the present payment system will lead to more hospital-based specialists and to higher costs of health care.

Various options for change have been suggested. In the main, they rest on the proposition that the costs of GME should essentially be regarded as educational, the prime beneficiary being the resident. One suggested option would have residents pay tuition to the medical schools, but then charge some appropriate fee for their services to patients. Other possibilities involve direct state or federal funding through education appropriations. All options have the same defects. Not only do they avoid dealing with the difficulties of the joint production process and the formidable accounting problems of finding and assigning costs, but they also would introduce serious instability into an already unstable and strained institution, the academic medical center.

We see no "one best solution" superior to present arrangements. On balance, we believe that the heart of the financial problem is whether the present patient-care payment system, which covers the cost of graduate medical education as well, thereby secures the lowest reasonable cost for patient care. It may well do so. The only practicable alternative to care by residents is probably for hospitals to hire staff doctors and to pay competitive service salaries or fees. We know of no studies showing that such a change would save money for Medicare, other third-party payers, and self-pay patients. In our judgment, the present system of paying for graduate medical education probably ought not to be changed. At the same time, there is great merit in the viewpoint advanced in a recent study sponsored by the Josiah Macy, Jr. Foundation:

> The costs and benefits of graduate medical education should be made explicit, and the financing of graduate medical education should reflect these costs and benefits. For the most part graduate medical education should continue to be financed by funds paid to institutions for patient care. However, if social, economic, or political conditions change, alternative approaches to financing together with their implications should be explored fully . . . What is needed is not a formula for financing but an approach. The key to that approach is an understanding and explicit recognition of the costs and benefits of graduate medical education. Although the available evidence suggests that, on the average, present costs and benefits balance out, our base of knowledge needs considerable improvement in order to subject this tentative conclusion to further testing and to enable the balance to be monitored over time.[28]

Important as the financing arrangements for graduate medical education may be, the focus of policy in government and in the academic medical centers should be on the substantive issues of determining the appropriate types and numbers of residents. Once these issues are decided, and the national needs have been expressed through government or other agencies, implementation will be dependent upon the machinery for governance in the academic medical center. Accountability and social responsibility will be expressed for all academic medical center functions through such governance machinery. Since this issue is of central importance to any complex academic medical center for all its programs, not merely those of graduate medical education, we now turn our consideration to overall governance problems and mechanisms.

NOTES

1. "Medical Education in the United States 1979-1980," *Journal of the American Medical Association,* Vol. 244,, No. 25, (Dec. 26, 1980), p. 2820; American Hospital Association, *Hospital Statistics,* 1980 edition, Tables 6, 8, and 10.
2. R. M. Gibson, "National Health Expenditures, 1979," *Health Care Financing Review,* Vol. 2, No. 1, p. 1.
3. Extrapolation of 1977 data in *Toward a More Contemporary Public Understanding of the Teaching Hospital,* Council of Teaching Hospitals, Association of American Medical Colleges (Washington, D.C., 1979), p. 42.
4. *Ibid.,* p. 29.
5. Council of Teaching Hospitals, *Survey of University-Owned Teaching Hospitals.* (Washington, D.C.: Association of American Medical Colleges, 1979).
6. "Medical Education in the United States 1979-1980," Table 24.
7. Gibson, *op. cit.,* Table 5.
8. *Toward a More Contemporary Public Understanding of the Teaching Hospital, op. cit.,* p. 29.
9. Gibson, *op. cit.,* Table 6.
10. "Medical Education in the United States 1979-1980," *op. cit.,* pp. 2820, 2823; Association of American Medical Colleges, *Medical Education: Institutions, Characteristics and Programs* (Washington, D.C.: AAMC, 1979), Figure 26.
11. "Medical Education in the United States 1979-1980", *op. cit.,* Table 32.
12. *Ibid.,* p. 2825.
13. Association of American Medical Colleges, *Medical Practice Plans in 1980.* (Washington, D.C.: AAMC, 1981). All the financial information is also summarized in "Medical Education in the United States 1979-1980," *op. cit.*
14. *Toward a More Contemporary Public Understanding of the Teaching Hospital, op. cit.,* pp. 42-44.
15. *Ibid;* Gibson, *op. cit.,* p. 1.
16. Council of Teaching Hospitals, *Survey of University-Owned Hospitals, op. cit.,* pp. 1-16.
17. Gibson, *op. cit.,* Tables 6 and 9.
18. M. S. Freeland and C. E. Schendler, "National Health Expenditures: Short-Term Outlook and Long-Term Projections," *Health Care Financing Review,* Vol. 2, No. 3, pp. 97 ff.
19. Health Care Financing Administration, *Health Care Financing Notes, Medicare: Inpatient Use of Short-Stay Hospitals,* 1978, p. 6; *Health Care Financing Trends,* Winter 1981, p. 8.
20. J. K. Iglehart, "Federal Directions in Health Care Policy," *Journal of Health Politics, Policy and Law,* Vol. 5, No. 4 (Winter 1981).
21. J. Hadley, the Urban Institute, ed., *Medical Education Financing: Policy Analyses and Options for the 1980's* (New York: PRODIST, 1980).
22. Institute of Medicine, *Medicare-Medicaid Reimbursement Policies* (Washington, D.C.: Institute of Medicine, 1976). J. F. Kelly, "Options for Financing Graduate Medical Education," *Journal of Medical Education,* Vol. 53, No. 1 (Jan. 1978), pp. 26-32. Rosemary Stevens, "Graduate Medical Education: A Continuing History," *Journal of Medical Education,* Vol. 53, No. 1 (Jan. 1978), pp. 1-18.
23. D. Rogers and R. Blendon, "The Academic Medical Center: A Stressed American Institution," *New England Journal of Medicine,* Vol. 298, No. 17 (Apr. 27, 1978), p. 945.

24. *The Graduate Education of Physicians,* The Report of the Citizens Commission on Graduate Medical Education (Chicago, Ill.: American Medical Association, 1966). Lowell T. Coggeshall, M.D., *Planning for Medical Progress through Education,* a report submitted to the Executive Council of the Association of American Medical Colleges (Washington, D.C.: AAMC, 1965).
25. Stevens, *op. cit.*
26. M. A. Fruen and S. P. Korper, "Issues in Graduate Medical Education Financing," *Journal of Health Politics, Policy and Law,* Vol. 6, No. 1 (Spring 1981), p. 88.
27. *Ibid.,* p. 89.
28. *Graduate Medical Education, Present and Prospective—A Call for Action.* Report of the Macy Study Group, New York: Josiah Macy, Jr. Foundation, 1980. p. 5 and p. 142.

Chapter 6

Governance of the Academic Medical Center

Academic medical centers, by and large, recognize that they face difficult and uncomfortable issues of organization and governance. All centers are increasingly compelled to make difficult program choices, to establish priorities among competing objectives, and to make decisions for the use of unexpectedly constrained resources, and to do so in ways that will best reflect their role as social instruments. Few of them have a decisionmaking structure that facilitates this approach.

The emerging situations in academic medicine demand flexibility and unity in decisionmaking at top managerial levels. In contrast, the governance of academic medical centers is plagued by rigidity of processes and a variety of relatively lower-level decisions that reflect the domination of multiple sources of funds, multiple centers of power, multiple focuses of leadership, and academic traditions that extol the virtues of faculty decisionmaking and strongly inhibit administrative decisionmaking. The difficulties of governance bear witness to the struggle among many contending forces for the conscience of the academic medical center, the outcome of which greatly affects it ability to carry out its social obligations for the present and future health of our people.

The exigencies of governance extend far beyond the task of uniting the teaching hospitals with the medical school. Each of these institutions encompasses a series of relatively independent operational units of substantial size and power, each pursuing different, often competing, objectives with more than one source of financing and control. Under current methods of financing and governance, academic medical centers function in centrifugal fashion, frustrating efforts to centralize policy decisionmaking. This fragmentation of authority for purpose, financing, and control makes it difficult for the centers to fulfill their social and academic responsibilities in the most effective, comprehensive, and balanced fashion.

GOVERNANCE AND THE NECESSITY
FOR CHOICE

The complexity of managing academic medical centers was succinctly described by Likert and Kahn in the report of the First Institute on Medical School Administration, sponsored by the Association of American Medical Colleges in 1963:

> Those who are medical center administrators face one of the most complex administrative tasks we have ever encountered. They are managing highly technical and different research enterprises; they seek to organize this research so that those who conduct it contribute their knowledge to graduate and postgraduate medical instruction and to the medical services of teaching hospitals; they are administering teaching hospitals and coordinating teaching and research into the highly technical services these institutions render. All these activities and others represent some of the most difficult tasks that exist in our highly complex society—and to top it all, the medical school administrator coordinates the activities of highly trained specialists who take a dim view of having their work coordinated in any way by anyone.[1]

Since then, the management tasks described have become even more difficult. Today the academic medical center must face significantly heightened expectations of accountability, particularly to the public.

As Likert and Kahn noted, many important units and faculty members within the center believe its overriding purpose is to further the growth of their own efforts rather than to delineate the role and size of each unit as part of an intergrated, unified program. Thus, the differences in purpose, nature, and size of the center's many component elements make governance truly a struggle if the center is to be integrated into a balanced whole—an entity that can be deliberately and purposefully altered as needs and circumstances change. This lack of unity and its overall social purpose distinguish the academic medical center from other large organizations in the corporate world.

The social contract between the medical centers and our society requires the centers to prepare physicians for practice, to advance medicine by developing new knowledge, and to demonstrate the optimum use of existing and new knowledge by providing health services to the public. In reality, however, this broad set of social obligations is developed and carried out through a number of distinct activities or programs, whose explicit objectives, expectations, and demands tend to be dictated by strong forces outside the centers as well as within them. The objectives and programs promoted by these forces are multiple and interacting. They are not always, however, mutually supportive, and indeed may conflict with each other, if not in theory, then in actual practice in the centers.

The problems and the requirements of governance are essentially the same in all academic medical centers regardless of whether a public or private university is involved. Private philanthropy in the support of these institutions, while still important, has been superseded by the vastly increased availability of public funds for both types of institutions, thus making the private, as well as the public, institutions increasingly accountable to society's expressed needs and desires. Since the public has come to view tax-generated resources for all social purposes as finite, the academic medical centers must join other publicly supported bodies in establishing priorities and making choices among their possible functions, traditional and nontraditional. This necessity to choose among alternatives produces great tension among all forces, both internal and external, public, private, and professional. The present organization and governance structure of these centers leaves it unclear who should make these decisions and what criteria and process should guide the decisionmaking. The significance of this issue has begun to win attention in recent years, as illustrated by the Commission for the Study of the Governance of the Academic Medical Center convened by the Josiah Macy Jr. Foundation, and the Organization and Governance Project of the Association of Academic Health Centers.[2]

EXTERNAL FORCES AND PRESSURES

Governance does not take place in a vacuum. Its suitability and effectiveness are tested most severely by the manner which it reflects and copes with the forces that shape the policies, programs, and activities of the academic medical center. The internal forces have been described in some detail in previous chapters. The external forces influencing policy and administration in the centers are government, private and professional groups, and the community. They include government at all levels, professional organizations, private foundations, national voluntary health organizations, regional and local community interests, physicians, and hospitals.

Among government bodies, state governments have had the longest history of involvement through their support of the developement and maintenance of medical schools in state universities. This role has grown over the years. In 1962, 85 medical schools were in operation; 45 were privately owned and 40 were public (state) institutions.[3] By 1977 124 accredited schools were in operation. Of the 39 new schools started during those fifteen years, 34 were state institutions. Thus state schools now constitute 60 percent of the total.[4] Furthermore, approximately two-thirds of the private schools receive direct financial assistance through state appropriations to assist them in carrying out their medical education programs. State government's major motive in supporting medical schools has been to develop an adequate supply of physicians who will practice in the state. In addition, there was some interest in supporting research to enhance the quality of the educational program. State financial support has been largely in the form of appropriations related to the size of the medical student body. In some states this included some support, though not segregated, for organized research by the faculty, generally as part of the rationale for the support of the university as a whole.

Starting in the late 1960s, some state legislatures provided additional funds to help improve access to health care for the people of the state. First, perceiving the pressing need for more primary-care physicians, some states voted special appropriations to their medical schools to set up and support departments of family medicine, the newly recognized specialty. In some cases these appropriations were made even when the medical school had showed no interest in establishing family medicine departments. Some schools, in fact, suggested that it was neither necessary nor wise. Second, an increasing number of states have furnished financial support for residency programs conducted in various regions of the state, particularly in family medicine, internal medicine, and pediatrics, with the expectation that many of these physicians would remain in the state to practice.

Federal expectations, interests, and budgetary support remain very large, despite recent decreases in nominal and/or real dollars. Starting in a significant way after World War II with support for research, the federal interest has since extended into the promotion of certain forms of health services, assistance to postgraduate training in certain specialties, assistance to postgraduate training in certain specialties, and expansion of the total number of medical students. Special federal projects have also directly aimed at altering the undergraduate medical education curriculum so as to interest some students in research careers. Other projects provided incentives for introducing the humanities into medical education or helped to prepare students for team work in delivering care. In the 1970s, federal legislation mandating the establishment of Health Systems Agencies throughout the nation required that each medical care institution, including the academic center, submit its plans for additional facilities and certain other special programs for review to its regional agency.

Local governments also expect something from the centers, because they usually represent the community's largest and most prestigious resources for medical care, particularly in large cities. The local demands upon the centers for emergency services, and for ambulatory care and hospital care for the urban poor have grown rapidly. At the same time, despite the advent of Medicare and Medicaid, the funds available to pay for services for the poor do not appear to be adequate and the local tax funding for these services is also limited. Nevertheless, the centers are expected to serve the poor simply because they are there. In addition, they are expected to provide care for complex sociomedical problems such as geriatric care, alcoholism, and drug addiction, which present pressing socioeconomic burdens to the local governments, but which have been high on the agenda of only a few centers.

A growing number of medical professional organizations also have expectations of and make demands upon the academic centers. At first, these occurred only in regard to the acceptability and the accreditation of the medical schools as educational institutions for the preparation of students for the M.D. degree. Such authority was first exercised formally by the state medical licensing boards and informally by the American Medical Association. The accreditation function has been carried out for about forty years now by the Liaison Committee on Medical Education, a strong and influential body jointly set up by the American Medical Association and the Association of American Medical Colleges. It directs its attention mainly to the resources available to the school, the organization of the faculty, the content and organization of the curriculum, and the school's relationship to its affiliated hospitals. The Liaison Committee Members and the site visitors who make the inspections are faculty members of medical schools, some administrators, and practicing physicians. Although it reviews all the educational programs of the school and its overall research and patient care activities, the Liaison Committee's major emphasis and concern is undergraduate medical education, leaving the review of virtually all the other programs to other more specialized accrediting bodies.

Residency programs for postgraduate medical education are each subject to approval by an independent national specialty board composed of faculty members and practitioners in that specialty. These boards are essentially self-appointed and self-perpetuating. They set the standards and conduct the qualifying examinations for their specialty as well as examine and accredit the training programs conducted by hospitals and medical schools. They review the resources of each program, the size and scope of patient care over which the training program has control, and the nature of the opportunities provided to the residents for clinical experience and related learning. Each board is autonomous and makes its own decisions as to the content and length of the program it requires.

The graduate training programs in the basic sciences conducted by the medical faculty must, of course, meet the overall graduate education standards and requirements of its university. Most of the impetus and funding for the growth of these programs, however, has come from the National Institutes of Health and, to some extent, from the National Science Foundation. These agencies have provided funds for research and for faculty salaries for teaching as well as stipends for graduate students. Applications for grants for these purposes are reviewed by a panel of outside experts selected by the government agency providing the funds. Naturally, the views of these external experts are used as guidelines by the faculty interested in obtaining support for an ongoing or new program.

Private foundations have had, and continue to have, an important influence on the centers. The support of the Carnegie Foundation for the Advancement of Teaching in the development of the Flexner report, and the role of the Rockefeller Foundation in implementing it are early examples of such influence. Subsequently, the Rockefeller Foundation continued to assist medical schools with funds for facilities and endowments for operational support, particularly to develop scientific research in neurology, neurosurgery, and psychiatry. By the 1950s, another large foundation, The Commonwealth Fund, began to play an important and continuing role in medical education by its support of activities aimed at paying greater attention to psychosocial factors in the treatment and teaching programs in medical schools. As mentioned in Chapter 4, it was this foundation that funded the study leading to Western Reserve Medical School's major curriculum changes. At the same time, The Commonwealth Fund also began to support experiments and demonstrations by medical centers in comprehensive and ambulatory care, which were new concepts then. More recently, as noted earlier, it has sponsored a program to reshape the content and shorten the duration of the premedical and medical education.

Many other foundations have helped medical schools either by supporting research projects or by establishing professorial chairs in fields of special interest to them. In the 1970s, the Robert Wood Johnson Foundation broke new ground by providing support to medical center efforts to improve access to medical care by demonstrations of specially designed patient-care programs, by primary-care residency training programs, and by special training programs for physicians to become "change agents" in the field. Thus, though their financial support of medical center activities is much less than that provided by government, private foundations are still extremely inportant in creating and facilitating opportunities for innovation and for movement in the direction of their interests.

Large national voluntary agencies interested in particular health problems also create opportunities for academic medical centers by supporting research and, on occasion, demonstrations of more effective and comprehensive care. The March of Dimes supported most of the research that led to the development of effective vaccination procedures to prevent poliomyelitis. The larger organizations, such as the American Heart Association and the American Cancer Society, obtain contributions from community campaigns which are used to support research, public education, and demonstrations of improved care for patients. Their policies are determined jointly by lay persons interested in particular health problems and by professional experts. While their financial capabilities are limited, they can and do influence academic centers by their decisions about what lines of research and what types of demonstrations of health care they will support.

Local and regional interests, lay and professional, also constitute external forces influencing the policy and activities of academic medical centers. The advent or the presence of an academic center is often viewed by practicing physicians as a threat to the size of their practice. This well-known "town and gown" conflict rarely disappears completely and can be quite severe; before one new state academic medical center could open, for example, it was forced to accept rigid control of the referral of patients to its teaching hospital. Except for emergencies, this center agreed to accept for care only those patients who brought with them a written referral from a practicing physician! Although in many instances skilled physicians in private practice in the community work contentedly and productively together with full-time clinical faculty members in the same hospitals, the prevailing pattern is more one of a truce in which both sides attempt to avoid open antagonism or rupture. Even though the leadership and the staff of the academic medical center are at all times conscious of the need to sort out its place in relation to other health service facilities, programs, and professional personnel in its community and region, the problems of competition for patients will become more severe if new public policies emphasizing competition in health services are adopted.

Regional and local community health interests will also press on the academic center, particularly the teaching hospitals, as a source of primary care. Community demand can sometimes virtually force the teaching hospital to undertake a certain program of care; this sort of pressure has led a few institutions in our large urban centers to develop programs in drug addiction. Like all hospitals, the teaching hospitals are also affected by a series of external forces at a greater distance. In addition to meeting the requirements of licensing agencies and the Joint Commission on the Accreditation of Hospitals, they have, in the past decade, had to accommodate themselves to the cost-containment imperatives represented by the regulations of Medicare and Medicaid as well as to the actions taken by Blue Cross in determining reimbursement rates. The emphasis on tertiary care and the development and use of new technology in the teaching hospitals drive their costs higher than those of other hospitals, naturally making them even more vulnerable to cost containment measures than nonteaching hospitals.

THE ISSUE OF BALANCE

The external forces that influence the mix of activities of the academic medical center promote an array of objectives that are often competitive, and may even be dysfunctional with one another. Policymaking is deeply and continuously influenced by these forces. The policies, programs, and activities of the center are not developed entirely out of the experience, wisdom, and dedication of the faculty operating in "ivory tower" academic isolation. On the contrary, discussions about present and future activities and priorities, whether in research, teaching, or service to patients, rarely involve only those actually sitting around the table in the office of the department chairman, dean, or hospital administrator. Always present is an assortment of outside forces, capable of assisting or obstructing plans or of insisting on attention to additional elements, which thus exercise an important and continuing influence on the decisionmaking process in the academic center.

We do not mean to imply that the medical faculty and the hospital leadership are always in agreement among themselves and are unhappily and involuntarily compelled to negotiate with the outside forces. Depending on the subject matter, different segments of the faculty and the hospital typically foster and welcome the expectations, requirements, demands, and fund availability from most of the external sources. In some cases, especially when the issues concern the number and types of physicians to be trained, the faculty may well join together to oppose governmental and other bodies. But this is an exceptional display of faculty solidarity. The objectives, programs, and activities of the centers reflect a large and growing series of separate social contracts. Each of these presumably has the potential of contributing knowledge relevant to health, enlarging the knowledge base relevant to the education of health professionals, improving medical education, or improving the care of certain types of patients. But as a consequence, governance becomes fractionated. The program of the center becomes merely the sum of such agreements, separately arrived at on different occasions, inevitably making the tasks of intergration, emphasis, and balance extremely difficult, if not impossible.

This issue of balance is crucial if the centers are to attain a secure financial base while directing their efforts more clearly towards the health needs of the population. If their programs and activities are to be in appropriate overall balance, governance of the center must be more than a succession of isolated reactions to the opportunities and demands from the outside forces as perceived by those faculty members who may be interested in a partiuclar undertaking. Ideally, the governing mechanisms should be able to develop plans that specify in considerable detail how the center believes it should respond to its overall social responsibility.

"WHO ARE WE AND WHERE ARE WE GOING?"

In a discussion of the academic medical centers in 1980, Wilson, Knapp, and Jones, staff members of the Association of American Medical Colleges, refer to a recent exploration of major problems of mutual interest to deans, hospital directors, and department chairmen. They specify the first of these problems as follows:

1. Medical center objectives must be carefully developed and clearly articulated:

    Who are we and where are we going?

    How can we preserve and enhance both the separate and joint initiatives of hospital and academic enterprises?[5]

Addressing the question "Who are we and where are we going?" necessitates concentrated attention in the centers to decide which are the unique tasks they must perform to carry out fully their responsibilities to the public that supports them. Clearly these centers must continue to play an essential role in education, research, patient care, and community service; the question is how their facilities and services can best be functionally integrated with other facilities and services to satisfy the health needs of their regions.

The governance of the center must address a host of questions. Are the different levels and types of education programs now conducted by the center all of equal importance? In a time of obvious economic constraints, which programs ought to be dropped or cut back? What criteria should an academic center follow in deciding on changes in residency programs that may be superfluous to projected national needs? Can this question best be answered by the centers themselves on a regional or national basis? If left to them, will open-minded decisions appropriate to the public need be made? By what criteria should decisions be made and who should make them, when the expressed needs for training in other health-related professions require access to certain types of patient-care programs which the center does not, for whatever reason, conduct? Who should determine, and how, the role and functions of different professions and specialties in the care of patients to ensure that collaboration is as fruitful as possible?

There are also fundamental questions with regard to the function of research in these centers. In certain centers, might the primacy and magnitude of research activities displace their major responsibility for education? In evaluating faculty, what is the appropriate balance between research productivity and competence in teaching or patient care? Does an excellent researcher always make a good teacher? By what criteria should decisions be made, and by whom, about the type of health problems to which a center's resources should be directed? Is it really important to increase the amount of attention given to research in the psychosocial dimensions of health and disease?

The manner in which decisions are made about what types of patients are preferred for admission to teaching hospitals has been discussed in earlier chapters. While there is no doubt that these institutions should be the leading sources of highly specialized tertiary care, is the present teaching hospital context adequate for medical education over the next twenty years or so? To what extent should hospitals or schools deliberately undertake secondary-and primary-care responsibilities? How valid is the charge that the latter types of care do not offer scientific and clinical care challenges and educational opportunities equal to those of tertiary care? How can the centers best arrange to deal with chronic diseases in terms of comprehensive care as well as research? Beyond the care of an individual patient, what is the center's responsibility to delineate and to provide for the health problems of the community, *as a population*? Should the center provide leadership in the development and implementation of comprehensive programs of prevention and care aimed at dealing with the community's leading health problems, whatever they may be?

Since these centers are powerhouses of facilities and skills in diagnosis and treatment, usually without equal in the area they serve, should their services be directly integrated with the rest of the medical care resources in the area? What is the appropriate role of the academic center in the region's overall portfolio of facilities and services? Does the center always know best? Who should make such decisions and on what basis?

Some of these questions are already on the agenda of the centers. Others are appearing on the horizon. The central role of the academic medical centers in providing tertiary care and in shaping the future of the health services system of our nation makes it unlikely that these issues can be shunted aside for long.

FINANCING AND GOVERNANCE

As centers face this host of issues, they often find that their governance process is gravely influenced by the external sources of funds and the strings that are tied to them. State support for the educational programs, mainly for medical students, is of a broad, general nature requiring only that a specified number of students be trained. Federal support has been of such a general nature only in the programs designed to help construct facilities for teaching or research and, in the 1970s, in the capitation payments supporting increased student enrollment. Federal grants for research projects and educational projects for designated types of postgraduate or undergraduate training set specific standards ad requirments. All suitable institutions may apply for these grants, which are awarded on a competitive basis.

In the past decade the federal government has made increasing use of contract funding, rather than the more flexible grant system. In the latter case, an institution or investigator applies for funds to conduct a project of research or education to meet certain objectives and satisfy guidelines usually set forth in fairly broad terms. If the peer review grants an application a high enough rating, it is funded and the recipient proceeds to use the funds to carry out the project in a manner reasonably consistent with the provisions of the grant award. Further peer review occurs only if continued funding is requested or if the performance under one grant is relevant to another grant application. Contracts are very different. Here the funding agency decides specifically what it wants done and often delineates in detail the type of staff to be used and the methods to be adopted, and sets a timetable for completing each phase. Furthermore, the project is continuously monitored by a federal project officer. In effect, the government buys the services of a group of university faculty members to carry out a specific series of tasks which it has outlined in detail. Thus, the grant and the contract are at opposite ends of the scale of initiative and flexibility for the responsible institution and the faculty.

Financial support from private foundations and the national voluntary health organizations generally permits a good bit of flexibility in the conduct of the project, whether research, education of specialized personnel, or patient-care demonstrations. The achievement is judged in a general way. External evaluation of these funded projects is informal except when a request for renewal is involved.

Outside sources do not always fund projects in full. Frequently the institution is required to match the grant to some extent with existing or new faculty or facility resources. On the other hand, the benefits of externally funded projects often extend beyond the achievements in research, education, or patient care to which they were specifically directed. In a flexible funding situation, faculty members can use some of the money to support other, presumably related activities they deem worthwhile.

Support for research has been the major factor in the growth of medical school faculties. Most faculty members appointed with external research support are eventually given permanent tenure by the university, which is then responsible for paying their salaries should external funds for this purpose be reduced or disappear. The risk involved in major increases in faculty size by this means did not appear to be significant as long as funds for research were rising sharply each year. The few administrators who thought it was important to address the question of the optimum department or faculty size were not taken seriously. This is no longer the case. As we shall see later in this chapter, the character and dynamics of the medical school decisionmaking structure make it difficult to discuss such long-term planning considerations effectively. Balance among activities serving diverse objectives did not appear to be an issue meriting serious institutional attention since there were many opportunities for faculty members, departments, and their subdivisions to finance expansions. The attraction of using outside funds to take advantage of these opportunities, even when these funds were guaranteed for only a limited time, has been very strong.

THE ROLE OF THE UNIVERSITY

The size and complexity of academic medical activities have created for the parent university a set of unique issues materially affecting its forms and processes of governance. In addition to the special problems inherent in involvement in hospital care, the university is confronted with major, highly specialized financial questions and with a demand for public accountability for its academic activities to which it is not accustomed.

Universities have found it essential to modify their traditional organizational framework so as to bring their health components closer together for policymaking and administration. Thus, over the past twenty years, the academic health center has emerged, representing an administrative framework that encompasses at least one health profession school in addition to the medical school and a university-owned or affiliated major hospital or hospitals. In 1980, eighty-six such centers were identified. Schools of nursing and dentistry, next to medicine, are most commonly found within this framework, but in some cases there may be as many as seven health profession schools, as well as several specialized institutes.

Universities display substantial ambivalence about the amount of power and responsibility that ought to be placed at the center level. Accordingly, the organizational form, authority, and modus operandi of the centers are not standard. A few centers, especially those located at a significant geographic distance from the other academic components of the university, are largely independent organizations, but most centers are much less so. The affairs of the centers tend to be under the general supervision of some form of special university governing group. Two-thirds are governed by either a separate board or a special subcommittee of the university board. Over 90 percent have a chief administrative officer (CAO) with the title of vice president or vice chancellor for health affairs, who usually reports to the university president or chancellor. The CAO is typically responsible for general policy, educational and service programs, and financial and administrative management. While the great majority of CAOs are physicians, some are dentists, Ph. D.s, or lawyers. About 10 percent also hold the office of dean of the medical school.[6]

The director of the university-owned hospital normally reports to the head of the academic health center, but about 10 percent report to the university president. A few others report to the dean of the medical school. In the case of affiliated hospitals, the administrator reports to his hospital board in almost all instances and only rarely to the university health center CAO or to the dean of the medical school. In addition to the health profession schools, two-thirds of these academic health centers also include two to seven specialized centers or institutes which report to the CAO. Some have as many as ten or more.

Even though the major purpose of the center grouping is to provide a framework for joint decisionmaking about common problems, the relationship between the deans of the health schools and the CAO is not uniform. For example, in about three-quarters of the medical schools that belong to an academic medical center, the dean reports to the CAO. In the other schools, the dean reports to the president, the provost, or the vice president for academic affairs. The situation of deans of dentistry and nursing is roughly similar. It is significant also that the CAO's office typically has quite a small professional staff. Almost three-quarters of them have no more than three professional assistants, reflecting not only the decentralized character of the organization of the center but also the modest expectations in the realm of overall center long-range planning, policy development, and administration.[7]

In most universities the CAO of the health center appoints an internal committee representing each of the schools in the center. Some such committees play a purely informational and consultative role; others are the major decisionmaking body for their center. The former pattern is by far the more common. One reason why some CAOs avoid giving the committee too much responsibility is the fact that the medical school tends to be the most powerful member, and could draw attention away from the needs of other schools. Moreover, a strong committee tends to limit the CAO's freedom to make his or her own decisions. In many cases, neither the CAO nor the committee has any decisive power.

The magnitude and complexity of the health activities encompassed by these university centers produce several unique policy and management problems. First, some problems are presented by the mere size of the faculty and the budget of the center vis-a-vis the rest of the university. In 1975-1976, for example, the total national expenditures of medical schools in universities without university-owned hospitals were 25 percent of the total expenditures of these institutions for all purposes.[8] In some universities, medical school expenditures are 50 percent or more of the total. The very heavy dependence of the schools, hospitals, special centers, and institutes in the academic health center on outside and uncertain funding, in contrast to the rest of the university, creates a potential requirement for additional stable university support. This need affects the overall balance of the university's programs and financial commitments, to the detriment of its obligations in other fields. Also, there are many academic relationships between units of the center and other schools and departments of the university that require coordination and adjustment at the top level of the university administration.

But the problem is also external. The top administration, especially but not exclusively in state institutions, is inevitably more exposed to and concerned with community expectations than the faculty, in terms of the role of its academic center in its region, its state, and the national health care system generally. This represents a relatively new problem for the university, for which it is not well prepared. The salient issues have to do with the types and size of manpower training programs, the effective functional integration of the center's health services with others in the area it serves, the optimum use of technology, and the center's contribution to health cost containment generally. Few of these issues can be settled outside the framework of overall university policy and administration. The university's role is often to achieve compromise between the outside public and the inside academics.

Within the academic medical center, the governance and policymaking relationship between the medical school and its teaching hospitals requires constant attention. A complicating factor is the fact that, in recent years, most of the increase in the number of teaching hospitals has come through affiliation with community general hospitals, rather than university-owned institutions. A recent study of approximately 70 percent of the medical schools showed that 30 percent of the schools were affiliated with five to eight hospitals, with another 31 percent affiliated with nine to twenty hospitals. Only 19 percent were affiliated with four or fewer.[9] Hospitals see patient care, their primary function, as the paramount and controlling consideration even though their involvement, often quite intimate, with medical schools bespeaks a sincere interest in education and research. The latter two types of activity are seen by the hospitals, in the main, as important elements contributing to the quality of patient care. This is in sharp constrast to the medical schools' view that the goals of education, research, and patient care are equally important and virtually interchangeable.

Maintaining a satisfactory teaching hospital affiliation requires attention to the needs of the hospital as well as the medical school in making decisions about faculty and hospital staff appointments, the involvement of patients in teaching programs, the appointment and supervision of resident staff, the scope of patient care, and the conduct of research. While the affiliation agreement cannot anticipate every specific problem that may arise, it needs to be clear as to how the shared goals of teaching, research, patient care, and community service, will be implemented in the decisionmaking process.[10]

The sources of payment for hospital services can have a controlling effect upon the types of patient care, research, and education programs feasible in the teaching hospital. As mentioned previously, the teaching hospitals are generally expected to provide care for patients regardless of their ability to pay. Public hospitals in particular cannot turn away those who cannot pay. To cover the deficits incurred, they must try to obtain additional funds from hard-pressed state and municipal budgets.

There are serious problems of coordination of services, particularly expensive tertiary-care services, among the several teaching hospitals in a center. Overlapping of such services is expensive, often involving extravagant and wasteful duplication of facilities and personnel. Since most of these hospitals are autonomous, owned and operated by non-profit independent corporations, coordination of personnel and the care of facilities requires difficult and prolonged negotiations among the staffs and boards of these institutions. Typically, joint committees or boards are established to bring the hospitals together for this purpose. Not all centers have such boards, however, and those that do have not met with notable success so far. A long tradition of institutional autonomy and competition in tertiary care and prestige influences these hospitals and their professional staffs. Another problem is presented by the fact that third-party payers, including government, are increasingly balking at paying for the direct or indirect costs of education and research. All of this produces difficult confrontations and conflict between the administration of the teaching hospitals and the medical school and also between the trustees of these institutions as they work to carry forward their programs.

The community general hospitals, which constitute the majority of the hospitals affiliated with medical schools, have governing boards composed of leading citizens in the community. Though the board is ultimately responsible for all elements of the operation of the hospital, it shares decisionmaking power with the medical staff. All such hospitals tend to be jealous of their prestige and autonomy, nurtured by a history of independent function before the teaching affiliation. The medical staff, consisting mostly of physicians in private practice, is especially concerned with the growth and autonomy of its hospital. This creates tension between the board of trustees of the hospital, its medical staff, and the dean and clinical department heads of the medical school. The task of the hospital administrator and the board of trustees in mediating conflicts and leading the institution produces many dilemmas of considerable difficulty. On the one hand, most members of the medical staff view the individual hospital's role in terms of how it can best meet their needs in practice. On the other hand, the medical school department chairmen and their faculty are concerned with how the individual hospital could best suit their academic programs. Solutions are often not easy to come by when these views are presented in sharp conflict to the trustees and the hospital administration.

THE MEDICAL SCHOOL

As the administrative head of the medical school, the dean presides over the full range of its activities. His responsibility often includes some twenty academic departments, the substantial, complex supporting services they require, and the overall financing framework. A few must also oversee the operation of at least one teaching hospital. Brief reference has been made in an earlier chapter to the increasing complexities of these tasks. Earlier, the dean's role was relatively uncomplicated. Operational funds were almost entirely derived from internal institutional sources, and the school's academic activities of research and teaching were on a relatively small scale, as were its patient-care responsibilities. External expectations and pressures, whether academic or related to health services, were also quite limited.

Today, the dean and his staff are involved in an enormous range of policy, procedural, and operational problems representing two distinct, though intimately intertwined, worlds—that of academe and that of the management of manifold services and programs. The issues that arise cover a wide spectrum from academic freedom to corporate decisionmaking and financial management.

The departments of the medical school are of two types, preclinical sciences and clinical, with the latter having patient-care responsibilities in addition to research and education. Both differ sharply from other university departments in the large extent to which their activities are financed by funds that *they* obtain from external sources. The average school has a full-time faculty of a little more than 350 members, with the clinical faculty outnumbering the preclinical faculty by three to one. Preclinical departments vary in size; some have thirty or more full-time members with tenure or on the tenure track. The clinical departments also vary in size, with the department of medicine being the largest, not uncommonly having well over 100 full-time members. The larger clinical departments, like medicine and surgery, generally are divided into a series of subspecialty units.

All the departments fund a large portion of their expenditures—not uncommonly more than half and sometimes more than two-thirds— from external sources for special projects and programs and, in the case of clinical departments, from fees for patient care. They tend to view these funds, which they have "generated," as "belonging" solely to them and not available for other school programs. These externally funded activities need space and supporting services, requiring institutional concurrence and support of the medical school and the hospitals, thus influencing the priorities of these institutions. To meet these needs, the faculty, in its many discrete parts, believes it should have a dominant share in policymaking and management. Intrafaculty competition and rivalries among faculty groups have increased. Within departments, although there is usually an atmosphere of collegiality, the chairman has a great deal of authority and generally makes the final decision. In the larger departments which are organized into sizable subspecialty units, competing priorities present special problems for the chairman.

The formal relationship between the faculty and the administration of the school is expressed through both permanent and ad hoc arrangements. There is usually an advisory board or executive committee, which consists largely, if not entirely, of department chairmen. It rarely has fewer than fifteen members and often has more than twenty. Major problems, as well as faculty appointments and promotions, are reviewed by this group. It also reviews problems of students affairs, curriculum development, and significant new programs, usually those that are to extend beyond the boundaries of a single department. It may also play some role in the allocation of space and some aspects of the budget of the medical school. In many instances, the relative role and powers of this committee vis-a-vis the dean are not clearly defined. Many faculty members believe that the dean should serve their needs as they see them and that his role is to carry out the majority decisions of the advisory committee. A less prevalent view is that the dean, having earned the trust and support of the faculty, should, after consultation, have the authority to use his best judgment. Most faculty are uncertain which of these patterns of governance is best. In fact, faculty members and department heads are, as individuals, not always consistent in their views about this crucial matter.

Direct access to the dean to deal with intradepartmental issues and developments that require institutional acceptance or support is considered essential by department chairmen, and often by the chiefs of the subspecialty divisions of departments. Although not all deans' offices are organized the same way, the dominant pattern, in terms of faculty relationships, is one that provides for an associate dean for the basic science departments and one for the clinical departments. Such officials tend primarily to act as the liaison between the dean and the department. Lacking a specific mandate with regard to goals and performance, they are simply one-way conduits to the dean and spokesmen for their departmental clientele. A small but increasing number of deans, however, have organized their offices differently, having an associate dean for education and one for research. So defined, an associate deanship represents a specific set of responsibilities for goals, standards, and performance, embodying the medical school's institution-wide interest and responsibility for specific functions and achievements. These deans can go well beyond the liaison function and raise questions and act on behalf of the institution.

Each school has a series of standing committees dealing with such matters as student admissions, curriculum, faculty appointments and promotion, and student evaluation. These groups may be elected by the faculty, delegated by department chairmen, or selected by the dean. Most committees ultimately report to the faculty as a whole. In addition, of course, ad hoc committees are set up by the dean. The faculty as a whole typically influences decisionmaking through general faculty meetings held several times a year. Because of the large size of the faculty, some schools have set up a smaller body—a school council or senate. This is usually an elected body which may include tenured and junior faculty, representatives of affiliated hospitals, and sometime residents and student representatives. Proposals for major changes in curriculum and admission policy are usually developed by appropriate committees and then submitted to these bodies for approval.

Faculty participation in the governance of the school focuses predominantly on the furtherance of its manifold academic interests and responsibilities. In the past, the concerns of faculty rarely included the problems of institutional administration and fiscal management. Currently, however, faculty are more active in trying to resolve problems of rival priorities among the many specific purposes and programs that represent the special competence, commitments, and interests of district departments and subspecialty groups in both the preclinical and clinical departments. In these times of financial constraints, these problems have become more obvious to the faculty and have put the present governance system under great strain. Much more is expected of the medical center's administration than ever before in terms of its capacity to handle the pressing policymaking and fiscal issues decisively and effectively.

THE FACULTY

The governance of the academic medical center differs sharply from that of the typical business corporation. The classical concept of university governance assumes that the faculty *is* the university and should make its policy, and that the administration's task is simply to serve the faculty and its ultimate social purposes by providing the necessary resources and keeping everything running smoothly. Hence, the governance framework is essentially collegial. Faculty members are not simply employees of the university in the usual sense of that term. For understandable reasons, they have a great deal of autonomy as individuals and as departments and subunits. Not the least of these reasons is that many faculty members generate funds through grants and contracts to support themselves and some of their colleagues, in whole or in part. This places undefined but real limits on the authority of the department chairman and certainly the dean. The authority and responsibility of the dean vis-a-vis the faculty, and that of the hospital administrator vis-a-vis the medical staff, are ambiguous at best. Because most decisions affecting programs and activities are made at the departmental and subdepartmental level, it is very difficult for the institution, as such, to give the long-term institutional implications of those decisions timely, consistent, and effective attention.

In the typical business corporation the hierarchy of control is much clearer. While professional and technical expertise among its employees is sought when needed, the power of decisionmaking rests with the top administration of the corporation. This provides the typical corporate structure with clear and effective means to examine its goals and procedures in the face of new problems or opportunities and gives it a great deal of flexibility in organizing its activities. We are not suggesting that the governance structure and modus operandi of the typical business corporation can or should be adopted by the academic medical center. It does appear, however, that the decisionmaking structure and organization of the academic medical center need substantial modification and strengthening.

Essentially, the top administration of the academic medical center operates as a loose conglomerate of independent units. It enfranchises groups of faculty members to carry out their professional tasks as virtually independent units. This independence exists not only because of the university framework but also because of the rapid and massive growth of the centers as collections of distinct, highly specialized activities, discretely financed through faculty initiatives, including, more recently, fees for clinical services. Since present medical faculty members developed their status in academia because of their professional performance, including their ability to "get grants," they naturally expect a large voice in policymaking. At a minimum, they expect the administration to expedite their work by giving it the highest priority, and providing the space and the necessary supporting services. And in the present period of financial constraints, they expect the administration to find additional funds or to reallocate existing institutional funds to maintain their several efforts, if not to facilitate their growth. A "we/they" viewpoint prevails within most centers: "We," the faculty, are working hard, doing excellent work in the eyes of our peers, while "they," the administration, don't really appreciate how important it is and don't help us enough.

During the years of institutional growth, however, the faculty of the academic medical center seldom looked to the administration for guidance and advice. The operative vocabulary of the dean was expected to consist basically of two words: "yes" or "no," with the distinct expectation that the former would be used much more often than the latter. The questions "why?" and "how?" were rarely expected or appreciated, nor did faculty members want to be asked, "Is there a better way?" or to be told, "Projects X and Y seem to be more important to our school than your project Z." This attitude is now slowly changing. Events of recent years have forced the faculty to begin to realize that their problems cannot be fully understood or solved except in institution-wide terms. And the mechanisms within the center for reaching such solutions are not working well, if at all.

At this point it is helpful to illustrate the context of the interaction between the administrative officers and the faculty at various levels. As stated earlier, about two-thirds of the medical schools are in an academic health center structure in their university. In a few of these institutions, the dean of the medical school also has the part-time responsibility of being the director of the overall center framework. In centers with a fulltime chief administrative officer, the job is often a staff position in the office of the university president, not a line position carrying the full authority of the president for policy and operations. A small number of centers are organized much more tightly. These are usually ones that are located at some distance from their university or in which there has been leadership, at the top university level, of a farsighted nature. Here the CAO not only responds to concerns brought to him by the units of the center, but exercises significant leadership and initiative, puts questions to the faculty, and initiates planning exercises and new programs with appropriate school and faculty involvement. There are other CAOs who see the need for this type of approach but are prevented from implementing it by the structure and the expectations of the university president and/or faculty.

The relationships of the dean and the hospital administrator are typically ambiguous and confused. Each official views the clinical department heads as an extension of his own administration. Whereas these two administrators look at their relationship as a partnership of two organizations, the clinical chairmen usually behave as though the medical school and the hospital are one organization. The differences between the policy and operating problems of the medical school and the teaching hospital have already been described. Effective administration of the teaching hospital calls for consistent, strong competence and clearly recognized authority as it develops and operates its services, at the same time providing opportunities for education and research. Medical faculties are slowly and haltingly beginning to perceive the relevance of this principle to the effectiveness of their work.

The tasks of the department chairman have grown in size and complexity. Key factors here have been the growth of individual departments and the predominance of research and its funding in the criteria for faculty appointment. The growth in interdisciplinary courses has resulted in fewer departmental courses, which act as a strong, unifying, intradepartmental force. The growing diversity of research programs within departments also diminishes opportunities for intradepartmental sharing as a source of unity. For the clinical departments, there is the added responsibility, often very large, of programs of patient care, which must be shared by faculty members with varying degrees of interest or competence in such work. Many clinical departments have become large, multiinstitutional organizations. Their educational responsibilities have vastly expanded. Some departments have grown so large, including a number of subspecialties which conduct their own residency programs, that they have had to set up department executive committees made up of the chiefs of these sections.

Departmental chairmen have usually been appointed bcause of their demonstrated competence as scientists. Many want to continue with their own research and try to guard their time for this purpose. Furthermore, not all have the leadership qualities needed to form people of diverse backgrounds and interests into a team to carry out the goals of their department and school in optimum fashion. The demands for research, patient care, and education are, under the best of circumstances, difficult for them to put into appropriate balance.

Today's fiscal constraints produce serious problems for chairmen in attempting to maintain departmental programs at their present scale and diversity. This is a situation for which none was prepared by precept or experience. The inescapable need to establish priorities in the allocation of institutional resources to the department's work, and to decide which opportunities for growth or new developments should be sought, tests the decisionmaking tradition within the department severely and, of course, raises questions within the department about the chairman's authority. As Robert G. Petersdorf has recently said, in a throughgoing and clear-eyed discussion of departments of medicine:

> Although the role of chairman has diminished since the days of the great professors—perhaps because there are no longer any great chairmen, only great committees—in most departments much of the character of the department is derived from the chairman. Though the Geheimrat image

has long gone, the chairman remains the pivotal figure in the department of medicine. I should say that not all agree that this should be so.[11]

For the reasons cited above, departmental chairmanships, which were once much sought after, have recently become much less attractive to highly accomplished and prestigious academic physicians and scientists.

WHO IS IN CHARGE?

It is clear that the system of governance of the academic medical center is not working well, at any level. In a recent discussion of the "managerial imperatives of the academic medical center," Wilson, Knapp, and Jones, members of the staff of the Association of American Medical Colleges, make the following statement:

> Medical school deans often find themselves in this dilemma: people outside the institution push for intra-organizational change, and simultaneously there are pressures from the inside to maintain the status quo and insulate the organization from external influences. In addition, public policy tends to reflect an oversimplified *ad seriatim* view of problems: insufficient directed or applied research, a shortage of physicians in some areas, and quotas for primary care physicians are examples of such perceptions. In this context, a group of university presidents observed recently that a significant amount of health policy in the United States is exercised through educational programs.[12]

The dilemma in which the academic medical center finds itself is compounded by the complexity of the internal tasks faced by its administrators, so well summarized in the description by Likert and Kahn quoted at the beginning of this chapter.

The present organization and governance of the typical academic medical center is not properly adapted to solving the issues that face it at all levels. From the president of the university to the medical school dean and the department chairmen, no one seems satisfied that the most appropriate and effective organizational framework and allocation of responsibility has been found. In significant measure, the uneasiness and frustration now growing in these centers results from their inability to approach, analyze, and evaluate the issues and develop solutions in an expeditious, openminded, and unified manner. The current structure and process of decisionmaking in academic medical centers protect the independence of their component principalities; they tend to fortify the status quo, rendering searching reassessment most unwelcome and most difficult to achieve.

More is involved than the fiscal stewardship of large sums of money.

In the face of shrinking funds and persistent external and internal pressures, the current form of governance tends to foster short-term solutions instead of the long term planning that is needed. Highly skilled professionals accustomed to autonomy and independence do not take well to administrators, even when they share a common background in terms of basic scientific medical training. The medical faculty, firmly rooted in the accepted and apparently successful traditions of the recent past, prefers to concentrate on its immediate, special needs. The administrators, on the other hand, cannot set aside long-term goals or the total institutional view and the requirement to ensure that the academic medical center will, in the long term, carry out its social contract as effectively as possible.

What is sorely lacking is greater certainty about who is in charge. Greater unity is needed in institutional decisionmaking as to specific purposes and priorities, the content of activities, and the size, effectiveness, and fiscal implications of all programs. If it is to carry out its social obligations effectively, the academic medical center must cease to be a loose federation of duchies and principalities. It must build a stronger institutional structure for policy development, operational support, and fiscal control. It will then be able to match and blend academic functions and social purpose into a coherent program.

NOTES

1. R. Likert and R. L. Kahn, "Current Research in Management and Its Application to Administration of Medical Centers", in Robert M. Bucher and Lee Powers, eds., Report of the First Institute on Medical School Administration, October 1963, *Journal of Medical Education*, Vol. 39, Part II (Nov. 1964), pp. 90-106.
2. "Report of the Commission for the Study of the Academic Medical Center" (New York: Josiah Macy, Jr. Foundation, undated). Association of Academic Health Centers, "Report of the Organization and Governance Project," (Washington, D.C., 1980), Vols. 1-4.
3. C. G. Sheps, D. A. Clark, J. W. Gerdes, E. Halpern, and N. Hershey, *Medical Schools and Hospitals: Interdependence for Education and Service.* (Evanston: Association of American Medical Colleges, 1965). Also as Part Two, *Journal of Medical Education*, Vol. 40, No. 9, (Sept. 1965), p. 12, Figure 1.
4. Association of American Medical Colleges, *Medical Education: Institutions, Characteristics and Programs.* (Washington, D.C., 1979), p. 7.
5. M. P. Wilson, R. M. Knapp, and A. B. Jones, "The Growing Managerial Imperative of the Academic Medical Center," in S. Levey and T. McCarthy, eds., *Health Management for Tomorrow.* (Philadelphia: J. B. Lippincott Co. 1980), p. 105.
6. Association of Academic Health Centers, *op. cit*, Vol. 2, "Presentation of Findings," pp. 6-7, 34-35.
7. *Ibid.,* pp. 35-42.
8. Wilson, Knapp and Jones, *op. cit.,* p. 101.
9. Association of Academic Health Centers, *op. cit.,* Vol. 2, p. 37, Table 5.
10. Sheps, Clark, Gerdes, Halpern, and Hershey, *op. cit.,* Chapter 10, "Affiliation

Agreements."
11. R. G. Petersdorf, "The Evolution of Departments of Medicine," *New England Journal of Medicine*, Vol. 303, No. 9 (Aug. 28, 1980), pp. 489-496.
12. Wilson, Knapp, and Jones, *op. cit.*, p. 106.

Chapter 7

Social Demand and Institutional Responsibility: What Is to Be Done?

At the outset of this book we set forth two important propositions critically affecting public policy for health and the organization and development of academic medicine. The first was that government can no longer accommodate uncritically the aspirations of academic medicine, which tend to focus primarily on the continued expansion of biomedical research. We pointed out that the public interest that emerged in the 1960s and 1970s after much political discussion, ranges over a set of health priorities far broader and encompassing than those that led to the extensive growth of academic medicine in the years following World War II. These new priorities center on the provision of equitable access to health care, thus raising large and basic political concerns about costs, financing, and organization for the delivery of health care.

Our second, equally consequential postulate was that an essential element in serving the public interest is a strong healthy alliance between government and the academic medical center, and an end to the disharmony and confrontation that have increasingly characterized relationships between the two parties. A more effective partnership is essential, we argued, because the academic medical center and government at all levels are now the two dominant forces in our health system—

government because it is the major provider of funds for all segments of the health industry and creates the framework for possible order in the health care system, and the academic medical center because it is the vibrant and powerful core of our increasingly organized and technologically oriented health system. While the significance of government activity has become well understood, the potency of the academic medical center has been inadequately appreciated.

We face the paradox, then, that these multimillion dollar enterprises, apprehensive over their academic status, are desperately dependent upon public funding for their survival and growth. At the same time, government is equally dependent on the centers for attainment of public priorities, and must demand, for the first time, that the academic institution it funds be directly accountable for performance.

CONTINUING ASSUMPTIONS AND PRIORITIES

In our attempt to understand how the academic medical center may best serve the public interest, we should now pause to look again at public priorities and constraints, and particularly to assess their continuing validity. For in November 1980 the political direction of the nation was markedly altered by the election of a new administration and Congress. Events in 1981 disclosed that there was sufficient bipartisan strength to support a pronounced shift of public policy from the liberalism inherited from the 1930s to a new political, social, and economic conservatism. While we would not claim to be capable of fully predicting the future, and many policy outcomes are still in doubt, we do believe it necessary to see whether the consequences of this turn of events markedly affect our basic assumptions.

If one puts aside the inevitable rhetoric of politics, it is clear that the new public policies expressed thus far serve primarily to buttress an overall national economic program aimed at decreasing income taxes, controlling inflation, increasing productivity, and decreasing federal spending and regulation, thereby hoping to promote the renewal of overall economic growth.[1] Except for the area of national defense, definite formulations of public policy for individual substantive areas of governmental activity have not yet emerged. Thus, it is only in the context of the President's Economic Recovery Program and not in precise social policy directions that we can appraise the implications of the sweeping fiscal actions taken to reduce federal taxes and expenditures (excluding defense).

The outcome of the Washington "battle of the budget" is very uncertain. Even though Congress basically endorsed the initial approach of the president to reduce federal spending substantially, continued high interest rates and a deepening economic recession have already led to substantial revisions of earlier fiscal plans. For example, the original objective of a balanced budget in 1984 has been abandoned in the face of unavoidable future annual deficits exceeding $150 billion. We can only assume now that the budgetary battle will be waged for some time to come.

As the battle continues, further reductions in rates of federal spending for social programs and a slower rate of increase in defense spending are likely. The stated expectation of the administration under "New Federalism" proposals is that the states will undertake a larger commitment to social programs, to the extent that they deem it necessary. But the fiscal position of the states is as precarious to forecast as their political commitment. Moreover, this expectation discards the principle of a national standard of access, quality, and achievement in the programs. In short, the eventual policy and role of individual states cannot be divorced from the broader national economic outlook which is influenced by inflation, interest rates, and general regulatory approaches of government. The outlook here lies beyond our immediate concern, and does not admit of confident prediction in any case.

Despite the sound and the fury of the battle of the budget of 1980s we believe that the central concerns of public policy for health care, no matter how approached, remain as we have described them in earlier chapters:

1. Equitable access to health care.
2. Intense competition between health and other economic sectors for constrained resources of a slowly growing or stagnant economy, leading inevitably to pressures for health cost containment.
3. A future surplus of physicians, coupled with scarcities in some geographic areas and in a few specialties.
4. Continued rapid growth and expansion of medical technology.
5. Rationalization of health services and high-cost facilities through regionalization.

Many studies and reports confirm that these are the major needs calling for public policy decisionmaking. Over 27 million persons, almost 13 percent of the nation, have no health insurance whatever.[2] Despite the availability of Medicare, principally for acute illness, this gap in insurance coverage together with the obvious demographic changes in our nation, will give a new dimension to the concept of equitable access to care. More than 2 million people are now over 85, an age at which nursing home care is probable for a large part of the population. By 1990 and 2000 this part of the population will have greatly increased, heightening the importance of access to long-term care for chronic illness and disability.

In September 1980 the final report of the Graduate Medical Education National Advisory Committee (GMENAC) estimated that by 1990 there would be a surplus of 70,000 physicians, which could increase to 150,000 by the year 2000, and that surgical and certain other specialties would show an oversupply of 150 to 200 percent by 1990. Even in the South, where total physician needs might just be met by 1990, a surplus would exist by 2000. The growth in physician supply will not necessarily prove very helpful to currently underserved areas, however. For example, the South faces the same nationwide problem of specialty distribution that brought GMENAC into being:

> The South has experienced a 2.5 percent decline in the percentage of primary care specialists since 1970. The vast increases of physicians in the South have so far led to increasing specialization in the better supplied specialties, rather than to an increase in the primary care specialties.[3]

Although the current administration in its early days proposed terminating the National Health Care Technology Center, Congress approved its continuance for a short time. It has now been abolished as a distinctive unit, but its tasks will be continued elsewhere. For as total health costs continue to be an issue of primary concern to public policymakers, the question remains how to foster the appropriate use of technology and prevent the unneeded expansion of high-cost and rapidly obsolescent technological innovations.[4]

The developments in the economy and the political arena fully affirm a continued high level of concern on the part of government and the general public about the containment of health costs. Whether cost control should or should not be given the priority attention that it continues to receive has surely by now become a question of idle debate. While such control was earlier seen as a minor issue for the academic medical center, the centers now fully accept that the total expenditure for health and the portion borne by public financing must demand their persistent attention—if only to protect their financial self-interest. National health expenditures have risen by 12 to 14 percent a year in the recent past, and are now estimated to rise from $287 billion in 1981 to $462 billion in 1985, and $862 billion by 1990. In that year, 10.8 percent of our gross national product would be devoted to health, compared with 9.8 percent in 1981.[5]

FEDERAL HEALTH POLICY AND THE
NEW FEDERALISM

Although Congress has adopted most of President Reagan's initial proposals for curtailing federal health spending, new substantive federal policy for health has not yet been worked out. Congress adopted few of the proposed permanent substantive changes proposed by the president. Still, we can be reasonably certain as to several features of the policy that is likely to develop.

First, while the growth in federal spending for health will be slowed, funding for biomedical research and research training under the National Institutes of Health will maintain a relatively high priority, as it did in the 1982 budget proposals. Second, consistent with its call for a New Federalism in federal-state relations, the administration will propose either withdrawals of federal support and services or decentralization of power and funds to deal with health problems, including those faced by academic medical centers, to states, through block grants, "swaps," and other means. Third, the nucleus of federal policy will be to deal with the issue of health care costs. And this is to be done by making price competition the fundamental strategy in the purchase of medical care on the theory that it will place both the consumer and the provider of medical care at financial risk for excessive demand by the former or unnecessary services by the latter.

While "competition" is in the best of the American tradition of free private enterprise, it is also clear that a competitive strategy will encounter very substantial opposition from many of the special interests in health. Unless the government withdraws entirely from the field of health, it will still have to establish the "rules of the road": consumer choice among competing health plans; payment by employees or government of fixed dollar subsidies to consumers including the poor and elderly; a set of uniform rules for all insurance plans; and incentives that encourage providers to organize into economic units that can function in marketplace competition. Paradoxically, then, any major competitive model can come into being only through extensive government regulation at a time when there is apparently a diminished faith in government regulation of economic activities, particularly on the part of the new administration.[6]

Our goal is to establish the framework of public interest for government and academic medical center cooperation, and we see no need here to enter into the debate on competition. But we must express our skepticism that a policy of price competition in the market can meet the fundamental priority of public policy, arrived at after decades of debate, namely equitable access to care. Eventually, such a policy of competition can only be implemented for those who have the ability to pay. At a time of resource contraints and a prevailing attitude that minimizes the regulation of providers, we do not see that this policy can mean anything but less insurance for those unable to pay and for those who represent high risks in health insurance— the chronically ill, the poor, and the elderly. Since, as we have pointed out in discussing the evolution of health policy, the public demand for government action in health is motivated primarily by considerations of equity, we do not see that marketplace competition can generally be the basis of effective federal policy.

The large question, still unanswered, is whether current federal policy will lead to a fundamental abdication by government of its past responsibilities or whether it will merely represent a swing of the pendulum of policy historically seen in American political thought. We are not sure. But the problems of public policy for health will still remain, to be solved if necessary more by state and interstate regional action, if not by national action alone. We do not rule out the possible resurrection in federal-state relations of Justice Brandeis's view that the states are the laboratories for social experiments.

Despite the political rhetoric, we doubt that any New Federalism can function without at least certain national standards or criteria on access to care and geographic and specialty distribution of physicians. In our highly mobile society only national standards can effectively govern equitable access to care for patients or the distribution of physicians and the approval of specialty training programs. Payment to providers will have to be under national standards, at least under Medicare or a hypothetical voucher system for the poor and those at high risk.

Regardless of the outcome on the federal level, the states have to deal with the problems of the academic medical centers, if only because 60 percent of the centers are in state universities. The loss of federal funds and the issue of competition are only a small measure of the states' problems with the academic medical centers. The escalating costs of medical schools and their associated teaching hospitals are of special concern. As pointed out in a recent report, even in affluent Texas, increases in funds for health science centers equaled the appropriations to all of the thirty-three other colleges and universities in the University of Texas system. States will have to address directly what medical education *should* cost instead of just supplying what the schools tell them it *does* cost.[7]

SOCIAL DEMANDS AND THE ACADEMIC MEDICAL CENTER—A MISFIT

Though the future of politics in health may be cloudy, the general thrust of the external forces pressing on the academic medical centers is not only cogent and relevant but reveals serious and persistent internal weaknesses in the centers which need urgent attention. It is therefore useful to summarize the picture of the academic medical center that has emerged in the previous chapters.

The pressures on the centers are severe and relatively new. They find themselves aggrieved, misunderstood, and subjected to new demands without, as they see it, adequate resources to meet these demands. They view some of the demands, especially those reflecting the new public priorities, as unreasonable and unnecessary. The most prevalent attitude among medical school and teaching hospital leadership today is one of "gloom and doom." Teaching hospitals feel seriously misunderstood and disadvantaged because the emphasis on cost containment hurts them more than other hospitals, and are concerned about how they will fare in a period of market competition. Most leaders in academic medical centers believe that the problems they now face have arisen because the unique and highly effective work they do is not really understood by the public and thus is inadequately appreciated. In effect, most of them have been saying, "Things have been going well, why doesn't the external world understand us?" It is as though something went wrong on the way to the future.

The problem for the centers is not that they may go broke or that they must anticipate steady-state financing. Their central attitudinal difficulty lies in their interpretation of stability. They feel threatened because they wish to continue to function as they have in the past, in a world that cannot be recreated. In the medical school, the central topic is how to handle actual and potential limitations or reductions in funds, an inescapable present situation and an unavoidable future outlook. The teaching hospital feels equally disadvantaged. In both cases the leadership wants to continue to live in a world that is gone. It is simply not organized or intellectually attuned to dealing with new social demands or with a new federal administration. If New Federalism significantly shifts the locus of political power to the states, for example, the private academic medical centers are especially unprepared to deal with state governments except in the regulation of hospitals and their rates and in financial assistance to undergraduate medical education through capitation grants or student loans.

We have seen that the 126 academic medical centers differ in their sponsorship—some are private, others are public, i.e., state-owned. More significantly, while they vary somewhat in program purpose, content, and control, they share two characteristics. First, they are not in tune with the new health needs and public priorities. Second, the implementation of the Flexner report on medical education, centering on biological research and the teaching hospital, still pervades both the medical school and its associated hospitals. The exceptions to this pattern, as we have noted, are rare and accepted only grudgingly by the accrediting body. Inevitably, the classical approach seriously inhibits the medical school from meeting the social demands made upon it. Similarly, it prevents the teaching hospital from adequately fulfilling its functions to deliver the range of health services appropriate to the population it is intended to serve.

While the academic medical center is not a single entity in terms of its internal arrangements, it is nevertheless an institutional complex more significant than the sum of its parts: the medical school, its hospital or hospitals, and the other educational and service facilities or programs affiliated with the medical school. Present organizational and administrative arrangements stress the independence of operating units as separate principalities or feudal duchies, a condition that has been fostered by the heavy reliance on research project financing from the National Institutes of Health and other sources. This fragmentation in governance has hampered the capacity of the centers to deal with the shifts in financing from various sources in recent years.

In our judgment, the public interest in health and medicine cannot be met by the individual actions of each unit in the academic medical center or, in its larger framework, the academic health center. The public interest extends far beyond the capacity of any single component to fulfill. We believe that the major defect in the government/academic medical center partnership is that although the center dwells partly in the university world and partly in the society at large, it is almost always controlled by the medical school and geared to the Flexner model of research and acute hospital care. The public has developed a set of needs and priorities, and government has introduced regulatory measures to which the academic medical center, *in its present form and with its present ethos,* cannot adequately respond. But government tends to construe the academic medical center too narrowly, thinking primarily in terms of the medical school and ignoring the reality that the academic medical center, broadly conceived, has become the core of the health care system. Thus, the academic medical establishment, whether acting through the forum of the medical school, the teaching hospital, or the medical center, aims primarily for its own survival. And so we have a fundamental misfit between the demands of our time and our political and social institutions.

MAJOR CONCLUSIONS

The misfit between social demand and institutional response

will be eliminated only after a long period of adjustment of our medical institutions—in education, research, and patient care—and in our political behavior vis-a-vis these institutions. We would begin the search for the remedies that will create an academic medical center to serve the public interest by framing a set of conclusions as guidelines for future action.

Our first conclusion is that we must recognize the academic medical center as a new institution and not a mere retitling of preexisting organizations for education, research, or patient care. Adequate response to social demands made by the public cannot be secured by separate approaches to the medical school or its teaching hospital. The emergence of this new institution reflects fundamental changes in medical education, research, and the practice of medicine during the twentieth century and public demands to assure society the benefits of these changes. Each country adopts its own measures for distributing these benefits, but all must recognize that the academic medical center is a national resource, central to the health care system. Thus, in time, Britain has brought the teaching hospital and all its programs of care fully into the National Health Service and associated programs of service. Similar action has been taken in other European countries, such as Sweden, Poland, and France.

Whether or not we adopt some form of national health insurance, we are failing to use the academic medical center effectively. Its great influence on the nature, distribution, and cost of medical care is not understood by government or by the public. For example, the medical school thinks of the community hospital as a teaching resource, but the state looks to the hospital primarily as a patient care and service institution. In fact, the functions are complementary and require a coordinated approach which is feasible only if the overall governance is unified. There must also be increased political awareness of the need for accountability for program performance entirely apart from the generally accepted stewardship for fiscal affairs. Although there are some indications of internal leadership towards making the required changes, the academic medical center is basically resistant to them. Pressures from the university and from government are essential if the academic medical center is to play its appropriate role.

Our second major conclusion is that the leadership expected of the academic medical center calls for a new mission for academic medicine freed from the domination of the Flexnerian traditions as they have developed since 1910. Despite their dissimilarities, all academic medical centers require a unifying leadership mission. We define this as *service directed at the protection and restoration of the health of the population.* In practical terms this requires that each academic medical center's activities be guided by a fundamental and continuing concern for studying, delineating, and addressing the health problems of the population of a designated area.

Academic institutions shy away from the word "service" but it is peculiarly apt to describe the mission of academic medicine. We see no difficulty in defining biomedical research and medical education as activities that serve to protect the health of the people who provide the financial means to advance medical knowledge and train the needed manpower. With the unifying mission that we have set forth, the academic medical center recognizes that it is a valid social instrument, entitled to community support and responsible under proper governance to balance its various goals of education, research, patient care, and— we would now add—community service. Only with a broad service mission directed to the health of the people can the centers behave as the national resource they truly are.[8]

The functions of all medical centers are generally the same but carry different emphases and are directed to different population settings. But we would argue that the fundamental questions each center should ask in its activities, including research and education, are first, what is the health status of the community, and second, what can the medical center do to improve it?

Our third main conclusion is that the governance of the academic medical center needs to strengthen its executive power and capacity. Greater responsibility should be placed in the board of trustees for public accountability. The organizational structure of the academic medical center should provide separate identities for education and research functions, on the one hand, and for patient care and community service functions, on the other.

Our fourth main conclusion is that the academic medical centers must develop adequate planning and budgeting systems that will strengthen institutional decisionmaking and priorities, increase flexibility to use and shift resources to meet institutional priorities, and relate short-term gains to long-term obligations. While stability in government financing is desirable, present and future economic conditions may make this an unrealistic goal. The absence of an adequate planning and budgeting framework, therefore, becomes a crippling defect in the present academic medical center.

While greater reliance on clinical practice income as a source of financing is inevitable, it exposes the centers to serious dangers. The first is a false optimism that such income can be large enough to fully offset lost or declining public funds. In addition, disproportionate use of practice income for faculty salaries has important implications for continuation of the full-time system which has been crucial to the growth of academic medicine. Clinical faculty may become so entrepreneurial that their interest in academic functions will be significantly diminished.

"Joint costs" will always be a financial fact of life for academic medical centers, whose funding structure will always be complex. Nevertheless, an important goal of financial management should be the reduction of ambiguity and the avoidance of hidden or cross subsidies. Undergraduate medical education ought not to be subsidized, as in the past, by research funds, lest the education activity be threatened with collapse as external research aid diminishes. No matter what the source of finance, costs for each program must be clearly identified and justified.

These conclusions may be summarized by the term "constructive leadership." In this inquiry we have continually asked how the academic medical center can best serve the public interest while guided by a new set of health priorities. We have pointed to the dilemma that, although this nation places a high value on the pluralistic character of the health care system, pluralism can promote wasteful duplication and inefficiency. The public interest therefore requires the encouragement of coordination and constructive leadership towards creating a coherent and planned system while preserving the most valuable features of pluralism.

The academic medical centers are uniquely situated in the health care system to take the lead by fulfilling a broad service mission. They have prestige, much of the capacity, and resources. The problems of ill health and of an uncoordinated system are all about them. If the centers would lead, the consequences would be substantial. First, the university patient-care complex would be brought more clearly into the community care system, where it belongs. Second, research and education would be closely related, but not limited, to the needs of the community at hand. Third, the familiar three goals of research, education, and patient care would now be supplemented by a clearly identified fourth goal, that of community service. This means that the academic medical center must give high priority in its teaching, research, and patient-care programs to the major health problems *of the population of its area* and to practice in the community. The center would evaluate the relative importance of different health problems by their prevalence, the amount of disability and premature death they produce, and the age at which they take their toll. It could then take the lead in developing service programs applying the latest knowledge and most relevant skills. Acceptance of this fourth goal would give such issues as geriatric care, alcoholism, mental health, child development, and arthritis the prominence in academic medical centers that they require. The implications of the service goal for the types of health problems addressed by the centers in their patient care, education, and research programs would be far-reaching.

Leadership cannot be exercised on all fronts at the same time. While activities under all four goals are interconnected, the priorities, scope, and volume of activities to achieve each goal need to be established on an institution-wide basis. Priorities and goals should be closely correlated with the appropriate organizational components of the medical center.

THE UNIQUE TASK OF THE MEDICAL SCHOOL

The unique responsibility of the medical school component of the academic medical center is to provide the continuum of medical education, from the M.D. degree to the residency programs and continuing education. Patient care, community service, and research are, of course, crucial to the success of the medical school, but many of these activities can be, and in some cases are, carried out in other institutions. This, however, is not true of medical education. For this reason, we believe that medical education should consistently get the highest priority within the medical school faculty, as a whole. Later in this chapter, we recommend a new approach for determining the scope of health services on which medical education should be based. The implementation of this framework will provide much greater assurance than can be given now that the commitment to education will benefit the full range of health services needed by the public.

Nine out of ten medical school graduates devote themselves to the care of patients in the community. Accordingly, preparing them for this work should be the most important task of the medical school. The interest and prestige that accompany the preparation of physicians and others for research and teaching obscure the need to concentrate on such questions of purpose as the ideal basic preparation for the M.D. degree, the total number of physicians to be educated, and the number of physicians that should be trained for the different specialties—in terms of community, regional, and national need. As to the relative emphasis placed by individual centers on their activities to prepare future medical faculty, we do not suggest that all centers should come to the same conclusion. But each center should make its choice overtly, clearly, and on an institution-wide basis, recognizing that it cannot do everything at the highest level of effectiveness. In general, we believe it is appropriate for a large proportion of centers to concentrate on preparing physicians for practice in the community, with a smaller number of them adopting, as a major educational goal, the preparation of faculty for the future.

Research must continue to be an important goal of the academic medical centers. They and the public should recognize, however, that as in other Western countries, much excellent research can be done outside the medical school. In our own country, an outstanding example is the intramural research programs conducted by the National Institutes of Health and by other research institutes. Our medical schools are not justified in assuming, as they do now, that the largest portion of research on health and disease can only be done well if done under their aegis by their faculty. Recognition of this fallacy would make it easier for them to address the question of balance and emphasis among the various goals of the center.

We suggest, therefore, that our academic medical centers need to clarify their goals and face the fact that, in terms of their social responsibility, the goals of the centers are not interchangeable. The goal of medical education should be given the highest priority in the medical school, which should view the goals of research, patient care, and community service largely in terms of their contribution to medical education. Such a position will not, in itself, reduce the quality of the research and patient care undertaken by the centers, but rather places them in an appropriate relationship in medical education. Furthermore, adoption of the goal of community service, as we have described it, will enhance the quality and effectiveness of the health services it provides and demonstrates.

A NEW MISSION AND A NEW MODEL

At this point, it is pertinent to put the Flexner Report into proper perspective. In its 1970 report entitled *Higher Education and the Nation's Health*, the Carnegie Commission on Higher Education wrote:

> The Flexner model, based on Johns Hopkins, Harvard, and before them, German medical education, called for emphasis on biological research. Science was to be at the base of medical education. The Flexner model has been the sole fully accepted model in the United States since 1910. Some schools have fulfilled its promise brilliantly; others have been pale imitations; but all have tried to follow it. It has led to great strides forward in the quality of research and the quality of individual practitioners. The Flexner, or *research* model, however, looked inward to science in the medical school itself. It is a self-contained approach. Consequently, it has

two weaknesses in modern times: (1) it largely ignores health care delivery outside the medical school and its own hospital, and (2) it sets science in the medical school apart from science on the general campus with resulting duplication of effort. This second weakness is now being highlighted by the extension of medical concerns beyond science into economics, sociology, engineering, and many other fields....We believe that the new interests in health care delivery and in the integration of science and other disciplinary efforts are wise. The simple Flexner research model is no longer adequate as the sole model.[9]

We are in strong agreement with this analysis. After seventy years and the development of new systems of medical care, it is time to lay aside the Flexner Report as the only model for medical schools. It has, of course, made a significant contribution. Its lessons have been learned. But it can no longer serve to frame the relationship between social demand and institutional responsibility that must be developed by the new institution, the academic medical center. As Abraham Lincoln said, "As our case is new, so we must think and act anew. We must disenthrall ourselves." Our academic medical centers should no longer be cast in the narrow mold of the medical school concepts of seventy years ago.

Some medical schools and the academic medical centers of which they are a part will have the desire, the resources, and the community setting to continue to follow the Flexner model. Certainly, not all academic medical centers need to do so, and they need not fear the unjustified intimations that their medical education programs will thereby become second-class because of their relatively low acquisition of health research resources from the National Institutes for Health.[10] Those academic medical centers that want to meet the needs for change and the new public priorities would move to a new model—the health services delivery model. This is the first of several steps we recommend toward assuming institutional responsibility to meet social demands.

This model should be fully integrated with all relevant disciplines in the university at the same time as it works intimately with the health care system, learns from it, improves it, and develops a new generation of physicians in this context. It would broaden the scientific base of research, teaching, and patient care by welcoming and fostering the intimate and deep involvement of the social sciences and the humanities. It would extend its interests vigorously beyond the boundaries of tertiary care.

We are reminded of the prescience of Dr. William Osler, who saw a serious danger in the manner in which the Flexner Report was being implemented. Fearing the consequences of the proposed conversion of clinical faculty to full-time status, he expressed his doubts in a letter to the president of Johns Hopkins University:

"cabined, cribbed, confined" within the four walls of a hospital, practicing the fugitive and cloistered virtues of a clinical monk, how shall he, forsooth, train men for a race, the dust and heat of which he knows nothing and—this is a possibility!—cares less? ...The danger would be the evolution throughout the country of a set of clinical prigs, the boundary of whose horizon would be the laboratory, and whose only human interest was research, forgetful of the wider claims of the clinical professor as a trainer of the young, a leader in the multiform activities of the profession, an interpreter of science to his generation, and a counsellor in public and private of the people in whose interest after all the school exists.[11]

With its mission as we have redefined it, the activities that should be carried out by the academic medical center can best be determined by putting its teaching programs and most of its research into the context of the health needs of the population. In this way it would be enabled to direct its research, patient care, and teaching towards the major health problems of the people in its region. The academic medical center would not provide or control health services for all the people of its region but rather would take the lead in trying to see that the concerns of the people about access, cost, and quality of care were met by the health care system. Within this context, it would be responsible for the full range of services of an identified population of manageable size, which would serve as the framework for its basic educational program leading to the M.D. degree. This approach would overcome the serious defects of the clinical education framework presently used by medical schools—a patchwork of highly specialized faculty members, whose miscellaneous interests may or may not be related to the health problems of the public they are expected to serve.

This approach is highly appropriate to the task of undergraduate medical education, which is to provide the basic broad grounding of knowledge, skills, and attitudes relevant to health and disease and an understanding of the major modes of evaluation prevention, and treatment of disease. The adoption of this approach would not, of itself, reduce the capacity of the centers to carry out their special additional function as the major regional centers for tertiary care and, in that framework, to provide postgraduate training, as required, across a broad spectrum of specialties.

The health service activities undertaken by the academic medical center would be those required to meet the health needs of the population regardless of whether they were for primary, secondary, or tertiary care. Centers would develop close functional relationships with nursing homes and other chronic-care programs and take a strong interest in preventive measures, whether by the individual, the family, or the community. This increase in comprehensiveness of services would greatly extend and enhance the relevance of the center's health services to its academic responsibilities and vice versa.

Because primary care is the foundation of modern health services and should play the pivotal role in the complex of services needed by the public, the practice of primary care should occupy a central place in the health services framework of the center. The concept of primary care means much more than it being the point of access to care. It also includes comprehensiveness: the capacity to provide the majority of the health care needed by the public. The primary-care physician or team also takes the responsibility for coordinating the special services patients may need and for providing continuity of care by assuring that all elements of patient care are connected appropriately. Emphasis on the practice of primary care also makes it possible to give it the prominence it merits in education and in research.

Taking this broad approach to its health services responsibilities would not interfere with the center's research functions. It would, in fact, have the salutary effect of inducing the faculty to broaden its research interests and relate them more directly to community needs. In addition, the center would have to consider the organizational and economic aspects of care and rationalize the supply of hospital beds and other services. It could directly influence the patterns of care for the future through evaluations, experiments, and demonstrations of how the full range of health services can be provided most efficiently. This is a responsibility to which the centers are not accustomed. However, it makes sense that they should address these organizational problems frontally rather than letting the structure of their services emerge simply as a result of the addition of a large series of individual, highly specialized, narrowly focused activities.

One particularly worrisome aspect of the current patterns of providing medical care is the role and cost of the application of new technology. Technological advances in medicine have been developing at a rapidly increasing rate. There are serious and difficult questions, needing careful study and evaluation, as to the appropriate role, conditions, and levels of utilization of each of these costly technological procedures in the diagnosis and treatment of the disease conditions in which they are applicable. Many of our universitites have the intellectual resources in their social science departments and medical centers to conduct such studies. The adoption of the health services delivery model we are recommending would facilitate research and demonstrations in this important field of public service.

We know that our concepts are controversial. Some will argue that the academic medical center is not a new institution, or that the medical school should remain in command. Others will insist that a service mission is inappropriate for the university. Others will say that our approach is antiscientific. None of these objections is valid in today's world. What we are saying is that the scientific capacity and the energies of our academic medical centers should, with a clearer sense of overall mission, be redirected toward a set of balanced priorities to meet the needs of the people and the needs of medical professional education. Not to apply the knowledge and methods of science to these professional and social objectives is to betray the public trust.

To most medical faculty members, the health care delivery model may seem a dangerous departure from their present situation, in which they can decide precisely what their patient care interests will be. Some may even see this proposal as an attack on their academic freedom. We disagree that academic freedom is involved here. The question is how the academic world meets its responsibility to fulfill legitimate social demands. The true issue is the institutional, not the faculty members' role. We believe that the institution as a whole, not the faculty alone, should make the decision to broaden the scope of health services and to alter the areas of relative emphasis. Obviously, this could very well mean that some faculty members might be dissatisfied with the level of resources for their areas of special interest. This is not new. The health services delivery model will, however, help to ensure that important health problems like geriatrics and alcoholism get the attention they deserve. It will focus the skills and energies of a significant proportion of the faculty on these problems. As mentioned in an earlier chapter, the assumption has been made in medical education that students will learn the basic things they need to know from their involvement in tertiary care. There is now an increasing appreciation of the fact that this approach leaves significant gaps that need to be filled by faculty and student involvement in other types and levels of health care. The health care delivery model provides the full range of exposure and involvement needed for this purpose.

The principles underlying the model we have set forth are not entirely new. They have, in fact, been adopted by a number of medical schools, most of them newly established, in other countries. This is the framework of the services and the curriculum of the new medical school at the Ben Gurion University of the Negev in Israel and of new schools with similar objectives that have been set up in Holland, Norway, and at the University of Southampton in England. In Poland and Sweden, national health policy has adopted this approach, and their existing academic medical centers are now turning their efforts in this direction.

SPECIAL CONCERNS IN IMPLEMENTATION

A corollary of our recommendation of a new mission for the academic medical center is greater recognition of patient care and teaching competence as criteria for faculty appointment and promotion. It should be recognized that, despite the rhetoric to the contrary, research performance is currently by far the most important consideration in those decisions. In addition to its effect on faculty morale, this deprecation of teaching and patient care activities does not help to maintain them at the highest possible level.

At least two measures should be taken to deal with this problem effectively. Only the rare individual is equally interested and highly proficient in teaching, research, and patient care. Therefore, as a first step, the schools should be prepared to recruit persons for faculty appointment whose special competence is needed in any one of these areas, without having to assume (or prove to others) that they will be equally interested or competent in the other areas. While the foundation of knowledge and skill for good patient care and good teaching are similar, this is not true for research. Because of differences in personal qualities, skills, and interests a person who excels in patient care may be much less effective in research, and vice versa.

The second measure deals with methods of evaluating capacity and performance in patient care and teaching. Faculty members believe that they can evaluate a person's research performance by reviewing his or her list of publications using various criteria, but that they do not know how to make an "objective" evaluation of proficiency in teaching and patient care. Many of these same faculty members, however, are not reluctant in informal situations to remark that a colleague is a "superb teacher" or is an "excellent physician at the bedside." These judgments are perfectly credible because, while they may sound subjective, they are based upon observations of specific activities and responses. Evidence can be obtained that is just as relevant in assessing the quality of teaching or patient care as the person's bibliography is in assessing research performance. In several schools where the medical faculty has resolved to recognize teaching and patient care as distinctive and valuable areas of competence, useful systematic approaches to assessing proficiency in these areas have been developed.

In Chapter 4 we noted the limitations of the present overwhelming concentration in the academic medical center on the biological dimension in the diagnosis and treatment of its patients and in its teaching and research. Significantly more attention should be given to the psychosocial dimension in human life and its role in health and disease. These aspects of medicine are not entirely ignored in the academic medical center. The major responsibility for them usually rests with the department of psychiatry, which, in addition to its work with psychiatric patients, gives a course on human behavior and carries out a liaison consultant activity with other clinical departments that request it. Social workers on the hospital staff are expected to "handle" the social problems of patients. Social science research in the clinical context is unusual and rare. Faculty members tend to take the pejorative view that the social sciences are "soft" in contrast to the "hard" biological and physical sciences. It is true that the social sciences face more problems because they must perforce deal with human beings as they live their lives, whereas the biological sciences can usually work in the laboratory with specimens and animals. However, the real issue is *good* science, and the social sciences have proven that they are capable of this, despite the inherent difficulties they must overcome. Most clinical departments simply fail to understand how strongly the psychosocial dimension influences the health of the community and how important it is in diagnosis and patient care.

The medical profession is seriously hampered by its almost total reliance upon biomedical knowledge and technology. We believe, as George W. Engel pointed out in a closely reasoned paper, that a significant cause of the present crisis in medicine derives from the:

> adherence to a model of disease no longer adequate for the scientific tasks and social responsibilities of medicine . . . The importance of how physicians conceptualize disease derives from how such concepts determine what are considered the proper boundaries of professional responsibility and how they influence attitudes toward and behavior with patients.

We further agree with Engel that the biopsychosocial model of disease "provides a blueprint for research, a framework for teaching, and a design for action in the real world of health care."[12] The future effectiveness of our health system depends in large measure upon the full recognition and implementation of this approach.

David E. Rogers has recently described this issue as the need to improve the "texture" of the doctor-patient relationship. He writes:

> I believe those in medicine must better use the potent therapeutic potential of the physician "caring" for the patient in strengthening what

medicine can offer to our society. Emotional access as well as physical access is important to people who consult doctors. Over the past ten to fifteen years, however, I have perceived a gradual erosion in this facet of the physician-patient relationship. The quality of the interaction between the sick person and the potential healer needs more attention by medicine today.[13]

We are not suggesting that the present situation has come about because of the callousness of the centers or because the medical profession is not interested in caring for its patients. Physicians do care for their patients, but typically in a manner that reflects the reductionist biomedical approach in which they have been trained. The practice of medicine is derivative in the sense that it applies knowledge from various relevant sciences. The massive concentration on the biological and physical sciences has brought great benefits. Comparable efforts are needed in research that applies the social and behavioral sciences such as sociology, psychology, anthropology, and economics to the problems of health and disease. This is not a new idea. It represents a movement which has been growing in the past several decades. However, except perhaps for clinical psychology, its growth has been much greater outside the academic medical center than in it. Medical sociology, medical economics, and medical anthropology are well-known and respected fields of concentration in each of these disciplines. But their role in the teaching, research, and patient care programs of the centers is still episodic, infrequent, and small.

A few medical schools have established departments of sociomedical or behavioral sciences. Social scientists are occasionally appointed to the faculty of departments of community or preventive medicine and psychiatry. Since many universities have well-established social science departments, it is prudent to seek ways of using these intellectual resources in the medical center. From the organizational point of view, it is not yet clear whether there is one best way to bring the social sciences into full play in the field of health. For whatever reason, however, they obviously do not now occupy their rightful place. They have much to contribute to research, to diagnosis and treatment, and to education in the academic medical center. This contribution is essential if medicine is to fulfill its potential and be optimally effective in the preservation of health and the treatment of disease.

Disease prevention and community health are two other areas that needs significant strengthening in the academic medical center. Health care costs are high and rising; moreover increased costs do not always seem to produce commensurate gains in the health status of the population. Thus public and professional attention is turning increasingly to the implementation of measures that will prevent disease. Our academic medical centers, however, offer very few notable programs in this area. While a small but increasing number of academic departments, mainly clinical, are involved in research and demonstrations of prevention or control of a specific disease such as hypertension, few, if any, academic centers have programs of prevention and community health that have a pervasive influence upon their goals and overall operations.

Preventive measures are either primary or secondary. Primary prevention consists of actions that prevent disease from occurring, such as immunization programs and counseling against cigarette smoking. Secondary prevention consists of activities to detect disease before it is clinically manifest to the individual, followed by treatment to control further progress of disease and prevent its complications. Screening tests for certain genetic diseases or unrecognized hypertension are examples of secondary prevention. Increasingly, preventive medicine operates through measures aimed at altering the lifestyle of individuals and groups as well as reducing or removing hazards in the physical, chemical, or socioeconomic environment. Preventive medicine is also concerned with health promotion. More than ever before, it is now recognized that certain crucial preventive actions must be taken at various levels and by certain professions, other groups, and governments, as well as individuals. Though individual medical practitioners and the organized medical profession are not able to control all of the factors that produce disease, they can influence a significant porportion of these factors. Furthermore, they can exercise strong influence on public policy in fields where they cannot control them directly. The physician can help bring about needed changes in lifestyles and in the physical and social environment by making his views known to the community as well as to his patients—as an individual and through his professional organizations.

The potential for disease prevention through changes in the lifestyle and the environment should not, however, deflect the attention of the physician and the academic medical center from opportunities for prevention through direct medical intervention with patients, especially in primary care. Hypertension is a good example. The evidence is now overwhelming that the initiation and maintenance of the treatment of patients with mild hypertension reduces the incidence of the complications of hypertension, as well as some of the arteriosclerotic complications, including stroke. The preventive effect, however, is contingent on the implementation of a full program of treatment, including consistent surveillance. All elements of the program need to be adopted by the patient: medications, diet modification, and avoidance of stress. The task is particularly difficult because many of these patients feel well and have no obvious symptoms. Hence, effective prevention goes well beyond making a diagnosis and writing a prescription. The physician must understand how the other elements of the full program of care can best be maintained in diverse situations.

Though more preventive measures of predictable value are now available to us than before, much more research in this area is needed. Such research needs cover a wide range of subjects, from delineating fully the human effects of noxious substances in the environment to understanding the problems of motivation in regard to cigarette smoking and excessive alcohol intake. Though the science of epidemiology is fundamental to much of this type of research, it is obvious that the biological, physical, and social sciences also need to be focused on these problems.

Institutional commitment to preventive medicine is weak. Many, but by no means all academic medical centers have established a separate academic department in this area. Some leaders in medical education, however, argue that since prevention is something that needs to be practiced in every clinical department, there is no need for a separate department. In fact, in recent years, roughly as many departments of preventive or community medicine have been closed down as were set up.

Most departments are small, often having the smallest budget and staff in the medical school. They are usually the most vulnerable when institutional funds are reduced. Preventive medicine faculty are often viewed as well-meaning "do-gooders" who attempt to proselytize others, but do not demonstrate their skills and effectiveness by performance in the field. While such a view reflects the general lack of appreciation of the importance of prevention among the rest of the faculty, it is a fact that most preventive medicine departments concentrate on teaching and research and are rarely involved in the actual conduct of programs of prevention.

It is most important that the principles and techniques of prevention and community health be given a significant priority by the academic medical centers. Certain fields of knowledge are generic to this area. These are the measurement and analytic sciences of epidemiology and biostatistics, plus social and health policy, and the organization and management of health services. Teaching, research, and service in prevention can best be developed if the faculty qualified in these fields of knowledge are organized into a department. From this base, they can interact with the fields that are cognate to their interests, such as the clinical, biomedical, environmental, and social sciences. Scholarly work in prevention and community health will, of itself, not achieve the educational effectiveness for which these departments strive. The department must also take responsibility for and provide leadership in demonstrations of specific programs of prevention in the center as well as in the community.

ORGANIZATIONAL AND MANAGEMENT REFORM

Effective management in a period of severe resource constraints will require the academic medical center to make institutional decisions that differentiate among its goals, establish appropriate priorities, and allocate resources to carry out these institutional decisions. The organization and governance of academic medical centers do not now foster such institutional decision-making and public accountability. We believe that fundamental changes are needed to provide for separate health service and academic organizations, more executive decision-making, and overall integration and accountability at the trustee level.

We have discussed earlier the interdependence of the goals of the centers. However, the activities undertaken to achieve each of these goals have their independent characteristics and requirements, which are crucial to their own success. Though many of a center's activities are "joint products," such as teaching in the context of patient care, one cannot assume that every element in a specific teaching program is necessarily best for the delivery of a high standard of patient care. We must recognize the basic differences between the management and financing tasks of the teaching hospital and other patient-care or community service programs, on the one hand, and those of education and research, on the other. We recommend a restructuring of the basic framework of the centers so that the large range of joint products for which they are responsible are appropriately selected and adequately developed, nurtured, and controlled by separate organizational entities. *We need the clear designation of two administrative and management structures of equal strength and authority*, which act jointly, where necessary, under a unified overall administration and trustee supervision.

The patient care and community services programs should constitute one organizational entity with its own governing board, management, and full supporting staff. Its budget should cover all health service activities conducted by the center, and should reflect the full cost of providing these services, including professional services, as accurately as possible. Initially, this administrative structure for the delivery of health services would consist of one or more teaching hospitals. In the course of time, however, particularly if the center adopts the health care delivery model and aims to meet all the health care needs of a designated population, other types of specialized units, such as nursing homes or organized home care, would also be included. Those institutions and programs that are fully engaged in teaching and whose professional staff consists predominantly of faculty members would, of course, be full members of this health service organization. A looser affiliation would link the organization to other institutions and programs whose involvement with academic activities is less complete.

In some instances, the full-time clinical faculty constitutes the entire staff of affiliated hospitals or services that would be under the control of the health service organization. In others, they are the majority of the medical staff. In either case, they would, of course, continue to play the leading role in the development and conduct of the patient-care programs of the health service organizational entity. In this health services context, the education and research interests of the clinical faculty would be a secondary consideration—but they would receive primary attention in the academic framework discussed below.

We do not underestimate the difficulties inherent in setting up such a health services organization. But the benefits outweigh the costs. This organization would provide greater clarity to the goals and objectives of the services that it delivers and lead to the strong management essential in this complex organization. It would clarify the strength and quality of the managerial imperative that must be satisfied if this complex operation is to work well. We believe that the obligation of this services organization to facilitate medical education and research can be most satisfactorily discharged if it represents the strongest possible service base from which to make accommodations to the academic needs of the faculty.

The responsibility of operating a hospital and other direct human services programs introduces very difficult problems, foreign to university traditions, customs, and styles. For private universities that own their own teaching hospitals and for state universities for which the state has built a major teaching hospital, these difficulties would be eased if the hospital were a distinct and strong partner helping to carry out joint responsibilities under the aegis of the center. Another important advantage offered by a strong overall health service delivery organization is that it could assume the leadership role in rational planning for the function and size of individual center institutions and programs required to meet the health needs of the area served by the center. Thus, it would provide not only the framework for reconciling the ambitions of the individual institutions in the center competing for growth and prestige, but also the organizational vehicle by which the center helps the community to define its health needs and the resources required to meet them.

Governance and administration of the more traditional academic educational and research responsibilities of the center also need to be sigificantly strengthened. Thus the strong health services organization would be paralleled by an effective academic partner in the center, subject to a common direction, as discussed below.

The present fuzziness and dispersion of responsibility for policy decisionmaking within the medical school hampers its ability to analyze its problems and options and to plan for the future decisively and adequately. The present modus operandi in medical schools does not foster an integrated approach. A great many decisions about policy and program are made at the department or subdepartment level without significant review at the school level. Although the expert view is critical in specialized areas, it is nevertheless essential that all policies, programs, and projects be carefully examined, evaluated, and integrated with the long-and short-term educational and research goals and objectives of the school.

If the medical school is to be an effective partner in achieving the four overall goals of the center and thus participate responsibly in the development and conduct of the programs of the center's health service organization, the position of the dean as an executive needs clarification and substantial reinforcement. Today, the role of the dean is seldom well defined. He needs to have a staff of adequate size and capacity to enable him to play the lead role in assessing and planning the teaching and research programs of the school and linking them with patient care and community service functions. His responsibilities, duties, and authority for this task, vis-a-vis the faculty as well as the top levels of the university, need to be clearly spelled out.

The governance of most medical schools provides for an executive committee whose membership is largely, if not solely, limited to department chairmen. This committee not only functions in a consultative capacity for the dean but also usually unduly limits his executive powers. Composed of faculty leaders whose over-riding responsibility is the welfare of their department, such a committee is of limited value for evaluation and planning to meet changing needs with highly constrained resources. To provide an executive committee suitable to the needs of the school, we suggest that it have a small membership, largely of senior faculty members, excluding department heads, selected by the dean after consultation with the faculty. While such a committee would naturally consult with department heads to learn their views, it would be better able to give the dean an objective and institutional point of view regarding policies that are not confined to single departments or that call for decisive change in the activities of one or more departments.

No ideal plan can be executed without some compromise or accom-

modation to circumstances peculiar to the institution involved.
However, it is much better, in the long run, to make these accommodations openly after the most rational plan has been developed, rather
than to build them into the development process of the plan itself. In
this way, after discussion with department chairmen and faculty, the
nature of the compromises made, and the reasons for them, will be clear
to all. This will be useful in the later evaluation of the implementation
of whatever plans are adopted.

A dean faces no more difficult tasks than those involving budget and
finance. In the corporate business world revenues, if not from a single
source, are nevertheless interchangeable, so that executives can make
effective budget decisions to back up program goals. In medical schools
such an ideal world is not likely to exist. Rather, financing will continue to follow the prevailing patterns of multiple sources and restricted
purposes. This diversity makes it even more imperative that the budget
be controlled at the level of the dean's office. Furthermore, the budget
should be divided into two major elements, medical education and
research, with specific allocations made to each department for each
program area. As we have already said, the cost of delivering professional clinical services by the faculty should be part of the budget of
the center's health services organization. On this basis, funds from this
source will contribute to the salaries of clinical faculty. We are, of course,
fully aware that most faculty, especially in the clinical departments,
carry out three functions in various proportions. This is desirable and
where it works well, should continue. We realize also that it is often
difficult to be precise about the variable time allocation of faculty
members to each of these functions.

At all times, particularly in a period of fiscal limitations, logical and
effective planning is seriously crippled if the institution cannot evaluate
and plan its expenditures on a comprehensive, overall basis. Accordingly, the school must be clearly responsible for the allocation of all funds,
including those directly obtained by faculty through fees, grants, or
other sources. A recent statement by Robert G. Petersdorf, a leading
figure in medical education with long experience as chairman of a
prestigious department of medicine, illustrates the kind of decision that
this type of budgeting facilitates:

> I have no objection to the general principle that the various activities
> of an academic department should pay for themselves. Thus, if the pro-
> portion of time that the department spends on the practice of medicine
> is 30 percent, 30 percent of its income should be derived from practice.
> Likewise, if 40 percent of the department's time is devoted to research,
> research grants should pay for 40 percent of the faculty's salary. But if

30 percent of the school's undergraduate teaching is done by faculty from the department, then the department is entitled to a much greater share of the institutional budget than is usually the case.[14]

At least one institution, the Mayo Medical School, has developed its budget on this basis from the very start. The clarity and relative ease with which the Mayo leadership is able to plan and administer the school's activities is remarkable and refreshing to behold. This institution is unique because its undergraduate medical education program was set up long after the Mayo Clinic had developed its programs for patient care, postgraduate education, and research. Nevertheless, we have found no reason, except the lethargy of tradition, why program budgeting of the same type would not be possible for any medical school. The clarification for planning that flows from this approach to budgeting revenues and expenditures at the institutional level is crucial to its success.

THE FRAMEWORK FOR ACCOMMODATION

We have argued that the research and teaching interests of the faculty should be a secondary consideration in decisionmaking in the health care services organization, and that primary attention to these two functions was more appropriate in the academic context, that is, the medical school. The principal function of a hospital is patient care, and in the modern, urbanized world of inequitably distributed health resources, the burden of delivering community service falls primarily upon the hospital and related patient-care activities.

We take this view, not to deprecate the importance of teaching and research, but rather to face up to the reality that in the modern academic medical center the goals of patient care, community service, education, and research are not interchangeable. In the academic medical center they are not held in equal esteem by all faculty, and they are not always mutually reinforcing. Since these goals, though shared, are distinct, and each is accompanied by a unique and changing set of requirements, it is essential that, in particular situations, the possible negative or inhibiting effect of one upon the other be clearly understood.

In such situations, we believe that a framework of discussion in which a spokesman for health services confronts his counterpart for education and research will make it more likely that the interests of each are clearly understood, and that accommodations are openly made with full recognition of the nature of the compromise that represents the optimum solution. This framework protects the center from the understandable enthusiasm of the protagonists of a particular plan. The importance of this principle is reflected, for example, in the public recognition that proposed research projects involving human experimentation should be reviewed by others who are not involved. In the organizational setting of the academic medical center a similar example that has been a source of controversy is the increased emphasis upon primary care. The typical university or private large teaching hospital is not a congenial environment for primary-care education and service. As a result, medical schools have formed more affiliations with community hospitals, a trend accelerated by the recently developing need of the tertiary-care hospital to enlarge its referral area in order to have an adequate number of patients.[15] Some may feel that this approach to decisionmaking by discussion between two strong advocates interferes with academic freedom; we would only reply that such a construction misinterprets the meaning of academic freedom of faculty members and disregards the fact that the decisions would be made by their peers in the context of institutional aims and standards.

THE ROLE OF THE UNIVERSITY

But improvements in the governance of the academic medical center must extend beyond the creation of strong academic and health service organizations, each focusing on its own academic or service goals. For the interrelationship of the four goals, the management of the intrinsically joint-product process of the entire center, must be unmistakably provided for at the level of the center overall. It is at this level that intracenter conflicts may have to be adjudicated and the interests of the university as a whole taken into account. Governance at the center level must assure that the policies and programs of the center are fully consonant with the educational and research interests of the university generally, giving due regard to university resources and to the jurisdictional interests or demands of the nonmedical components.

In the past decade, two major reports have made recommendations regarding the governance of the academic medical center. These are the Report of the Commission for the Study of the Governance of the Academic Medical Center, sponsored by the Josiah Macy Jr. Foundation in the early 1970s, and the Report of the Organization and Governance Project of the Association of Academic Health Centers, in 1980.[16] While these recommendations do not compel agreement in all quarters, they should command serious attention.

Since our universities do not all have the same orientation and objectives and since they have varied private and public sponsorship, no uniform plan of organization and governance of academic medical centers will be suitable for all universities. Some medical centers, like those embracing the Harvard Medical School or the College of Physicians and Surgeons of Columbia University, are quite distinct organizations with a very loose relationship with the university in terms of academic and fiscal policies. Others, like those of the University of Chicago and Stanford University are intimately intergrated with the university. Most centers are somewhere in between. Nevertheless, certain principles should be applied in all cases.

First, the university should create an identifiable unit at the top university level to manage all the components of the academic medical center and to coordinate its activities with the society at large. Second, this unit should be headed by a chief administrative officer who can speak and act authoritatively for the university. This officer should not also be the dean of the medical school or any other university component. Third, the chief administrative officer should be assisted by a small joint advisory board to bring together the academic and health service units. Fourth, and probably most important, the medical center should be guided by a clear statement of mission, goals, and specific program objectives, reflecting the aims of the university and the associated hospitals and service units and a coordinated perception of institutional responsibility to social demands. Leadership to develop and maintain this mission statement should rest with the chief administrative officer. Finally, the chief administrative officer of the center requires a strong staff to support him in programmatic and managerial activities, including fiscal, for which university responsibility is essential. The appropriate size of this staff and its power of decision will depend on the university involved.

ACCOUNTABILITY AND THE ROLE OF THE TRUSTEES

Decisionmaking and conflict resolution in the academic medical center is ultimately the responsibility of a board of trustees of the university, academic medical center, or hospital. In a formal or legal sense, the authority of a board to govern the institution involved is virtually absolute, and court decisions affirm the legal liability of boards of trustees. But reality and law are not always synonymous, especially where the laity and the professions come together, as in the academic medical center or the hospital. In these situations, the layman may be easily confounded by medical experts and find himself incapable of dealing with the internal power politics of the institutions; the board then tends to become a "rubber stamp" for the administration, a luxury that boards can no longer afford.

The pressure of external forces upon the academic medical center—whether evidenced as community demands for service, federal or state regulations, policies for cost containment, diminished funding for research, or any of the other ways we have discussed—requires that the board of trustees be the court of last resort for decisionmaking and goal-setting. Trustees, selected on a broadly representative basis, cannot serve as advocates of special groups with vested interests in the institution. Their concern has to be to serve the general welfare of the entire institution and through this outlook to see that the institution performs optimally on behalf of society.[17]

When university administrators and faculty contend with government about matters of accountability, their acrimonious disputes and confrontations tend to be about *financial* and *administrative* accountability, which is generally supposed to be established through evidence of financial propriety.[18] Despite some governmental concern from time to time, it has generally been accepted that *scientific* accountability is appropriately handled by peer review mechanisms. But accountability is a popular, yet elusive, concept of many meanings. It clearly connotes obligation—scientific, financial, or social. Thus it necessarily raises the questions of the means of accountability, to whom the accountability is expressed, and to whom accountability is owed.[19]

We are here concerned with social and performance accountability, which emphasizes outcome and goal achievement, or to express it even more succinctly, the public interest. If we expect the academic medical center to be fully responsive to the public interest, we must ask the boards of trustees to be actively engaged in helping achieve the necessary program balance and the appropriate allocation of resources devoted to the quality of education, advancement of medical knowledge, and improvement in the health status of the public. The medical faculty and medical center administration usually address only one part of the issue, namely the need for better public understanding of medicine and science. Equally important, however, is a better understanding by the academic community of their responsibility to society for applying scientific knowledge to protect and restore the health of the public. It is a major task of the trustees to bring this understanding to the academic community.

Scientific accountability lies in the realm of academic review; fiscal accountability lies in the administrative structure and regulations; and assurance of quality of care is the obligation of the medical profession. But social accountability, or the public interest, is to be assured by the trustees as their own inescapable obligation.

The wise use of science depends on value judgements, in which the public has the most at stake. Although it is appropriate for trustees to honor the expertise of faculty, they must deepen their own understanding of the scientific and social issues on which they are asked to decide. There is convincing evidence in medicine, as well as in other scientific and technical fields, that representative, intelligent lay persons can indeed understand the underlying nature of the issues, and that they bring a unique and vital quality to such discussions. The question a trustee fears is naive, may be most penetrating. The major policy decisions in the centers cannot and should not be made by the professionals alone. Participation by the community would be greatly strengthened by the deliberate demystification of the work, problems, and potential of the expert professionals. Modifying and strengthening the role and activities of the trustees as we have suggested will help them carry out their responsibility to guide the institution so that it can best serve the public which supports it.

THE RESPONSIBILITY OF GOVERNMENT AND PUBLIC UNDERSTANDING

We cannot expect that the academic medical center will pursue the public interest without an active role by government and clear political action to support it. Academic medical centers have had reason to doubt the extent and the stability of past political commitments. Consequently, they will not readily change direction without strong, continuing external pressure.

Here we have to ask whether the theory and practice of political pluralism, as it has been known in the past, can truly serve the public interest in a future of unexpectedly and substantially constrained resources. Public policymaking in health has given great weight to the power of the special interests of hospitals, medical schools, organized medicine, third-party payers, and the other institutional participants in the health industry. Political decisions have tended to ratify the outcome of pluralistic bargaining on the assumption that there has been professional consensus among individuals and organizations that promotion of the public good is their principal goal. Actually, as we have seen, self-fulfillment and survival are equally operative institutional goals.[20]

Given the economic outlook, the system of pluralistic bargaining is even less likely to lead to appropriate answers in the future. We must set aside "the myth of the automatic society granted us by an all-encompassing, ideally self-correcting, providentially automatic political process."[21]

The dilemma is that we ascribe high value to the processes of pluralism, as we have pointed out. This value, seemingly ever more popular, underpins the apparent preference to develop a health strategy based on competition. Much depends on the format of the competitive scheme. We disagree, as we have indicated, with the so-called competitive solution. But in any case, if government expects the academic medical center to change direction to meet the public interest, special provision needs to be made for the higher average costs in teaching hospitals, small and large. These costs are related to undergraduate and postgaduate medical education and allied health training, research applications and tertiary care, payment for the poor, and organized ambulatory care in academic medical center hospitals.

Efforts to institute a competitive strategy are likely to founder. Society must still develop public policies for health that promote and support the mission and operations of the academic medical center. We see the continuing need for policies in at least four major areas:

First, the present commitment to a reasonable and stable level of government funding for biomedical research and training is fundamental. Without such assurance, we cannot expect the academic underpinning necessary for the further development of health care, not to mention a new direction.

Second, government must assure the medical centers that they can expect reasonable payment for the services they provide. While the current political condition obviously has pushed aside the debate on national health insurance, the social demands for care remain a real pressure upon the medical centers. An adequate payments policy for primary care is especially required.

Third, it is important to find ways of financing graduate medical education and controlling the numbers and types of specialists. As a political matter, we would doubt that financing proposals to move funds from patient care to education appropriations can succeed. More critical than the shift of funds are the manpower decisions and the selection of institutional mechanisms of control, e.g., specialty boards or government agencies.

Finally, at either the federal or the state level, government must provide for effective health planning and regionalization of facilities and services. The academic medical center has special needs that must be taken into account, but by the same token, such planning and regionalization must assure that the facilities and services of the academic medical center are fully and economically integrated with those of its region as a whole.

In the end, government must be prepared to make specific performance demands upon the academic medical center, since outside forces are needed to compel change (just as the Flexner Report of 1910 was an outside force). State as well as federal government should assure the capacity of academic medicine to serve the public interest and should overcome its reluctance to monitor the performance of the academic medical center in meeting its stated goals.

In a democratic society, government cannot undertake fundamental changes without broad public understanding of the issues and support for the suggested changes. Although it may be difficult to build public understanding of the academic medical center, a long-term program of political education is essential. The academic medical center will no longer be a mystery if the public knows what it is, what role it plays in the health care system, and what it wants the center to do.

The inescapable fact—for the citizen, the academic medical center, and government—is that the centers must be openly accountable to the public, which pays the bill through taxes, health insurance premiums, and fees. We have no blueprint for a political educational program to awaken the public to the magnitude of its financial stake and its dependence upon the academic medical center. We do believe that such a program should begin, close to the people, at the community level. One step would be to heighten citizens' understanding that the center has a major influence on the quality, effectiveness, and cost of their health care. Another step would be to make the public aware that it pays for virtually everything that the centers do, and thus can legitimately demand that they serve community interests.

Public understanding, once developed, can be brought to bear upon a number of influential groups. Clearly, local, state, and federal legislators and executives are important channels and contacts for the public. But citizens can also make themselves heard through their participation in local and regional health planning. Finally, the boards of trustees of the academic medical centers, however they are organized, need to be in direct contact with the public. Furthermore, they should take responsibility for seeing that the faculty and other professionals in the medical centers honor their social contract with the public. For it is only by honoring this social contract that the academic medical center's activities will be consonant with the public interest.

NOTES

1. The White House, *A Program for Economic Recovery*, February 18, 1981.
2. National Center for Health Services Research, *"Who Are the Uninsured?"* Data Preview 1 from the National Health Care Expenditure Study, Public Health Service,

Department of Health and Human Services (Washington, D.C., 1980).

3. H. L. McPheeters, M.D., ed., *Alternatives in Medical Education in the South; Supply, Distribution, and Cost.* a report of a regional conference in Atlanta, December 1980 (Atlanta: Southern Regional Education Board, 1981), p.11.

4. S. A. Schroeder, "Medical Technology and Academic Medicine: The Doctor-Producers' Dilemma." *Journal of Medical Education,* Vol. 56, No. 8 (Aug. 1981), pp. 634-639.

5. M. S. Freeland and C. E. Schendler, "National Health Expenditures: Short-Term Outlook and Long-Term Projections," *Health Care Financing Review* (Winter 1981), p. 977.

6. John K. Iglehart, "Drawing the Lines for the Debate on Competition," *New England Journal of Medicine,* Vol. 305 (1981), pp. 291-296; A. C. Enthoven, "The Competition Strategy: Status and Prospects," *New England Journal of Medicine,* Vol. 304 (1981), pp. 109-112.

7. H. L. McPheeters, *op. cit.* pp. 33-34.

8. R. Heyssel, "The Role of the Urban University Medical Center," in E. Ginzberg and A. M. Yohalen, eds., *The University Medical Center and the Metropolis,* (New York: Josiah Macy, Jr. Foundation, 1974), pp. 35-38.

9. Carnegie Commission on Higher Education, *Higher Education and the Nation's Health* (New York: McGraw-Hill, 1980), pp. 3-5.

10. D. R. Perry, D. R. Challoner, and R. J. Oberst, "Research Advances and Resource Constraints," *New England Journal of Medicine,* Vol. 305, No. 6 (1981) pp. 320-324.

11. Quoted in J. P. McGovern and C. G. Roland, *William Osler: The Continuing Education* (Springfield: Charles Thomas, 1969), p. 303.

12. G. L. Engel, "The Need for a New Medical Model: A Challenge for Biomedicine," *Science,* Vol. 196, No. 4286 (1977), pp. 129-135.

13. D. E. Rogers, *American Medicine: Challenges for the 1980's* (Cambridge: Ballinger, 1978), p. 53.

14. R. G. Petersdorf, "The Evolution of Departments of Medicine," *New England Journal of Medicine,* Vol. 303, No. 9 (Aug. 28, 1980), p. 495.

15. J. Z. Bowers, and E. F. Purcell, eds. *The University and Medicine, The Past, The Present, and Tomorrow* (New York: Josiah Macy, Jr. Foundation, 1977), p. 157.

16. *Report of the Commission for the Study of the Governance of the Academic Medical Center.* (New York: Josiah Macy, Jr. Foundation, undated). See also Association of Academic Health Centers, *Report of the Organization and Governance Project* (Washington, D.C., April 1980), pp. 115-125.

17. R. N. Witcoff, "The Present Influence and Future Role of Boards of Trustees on the Organization and Governance of Academic Health Centers," in Association of Academic Health Centers, *op. cit.,* Vol. 3, pp. 143-151.

18. National Commission on Research, *Accountability: Restoring the Quality of the Partnership.* (Washington, D.C.: National Commission on Research, 1980).

19. H. C. Mansfield, "The Quest for Accountability," *Public Administration Review,* Vol. 41, No. 3 (May-June 1981), p. 397.

20. C. Taft and S. Levine, "Problems of Federal Policies and Strategies to Influence the Quality of Health Care," in R. H. Egdahl and P. M. Gertman, *Quality Assurance in Health Care* (Germantown, Md.: Aspen Systems, 1976), pp. 31-57.

21. T. Lowi, *The End of Liberalism: Ideology, Policy, and the Crisis of Public Authority* (New York: W. W. Norton and Co., 1969), p. 54.

Index

A

Academic health center, use of term, 44
Academic medical center, 43–76
  access to, 86–87
  as big business, 164–165
  business management of, 11
  community service and, 67, 68–69,
    227–228
  component institutions in, 9–10
  conclusions concerning, 224–228
  coordination of services in, 206
  costs and, 87–89, 164–165
  current status of, 58–61
  definition and concepts in, 43–45
  delivery of health services and, 83–84
  department chairmen and, 212–213
  deregulation and competition in, 96–98
  as dominant force in health care system,
    217–218
  expenditures of, 51–52, 164–165
  faculty practice plans in, 89–91,
    94–96, 226–227
  federal support for, 52–53, 60
  financial problems with, 10
  Flexnerian traditions and, 225–226
  future directions for, 73–76, 199–201
  governance of, 181–214, 224, 226
  government and, 10, 11–12
  health care costs and, 91–92
  health planning and regionalization and,
    101–106
  health services delivery model in,
    231–234
  Health Systems Agencies (HSA) and,
    101–102
  hospital-medical school relationships and,
    61–66
  increasing growth and influence of, 51–54
  as new institution, 225
  new model needed in, 229–234
  new technology and, 232–233
  patient care in, 79–80, 154–155
  physician oversupply and, 70
  planning and budget systems in, 226–227
  preventive medicine and, 236–239
  primary care and, 98–101, 232
  problems facing, 71–73
  program goals of, 66–73
  public accountability of, 59
  public policy and, 39, 73–75, 89
  reforms needed in, 155–157
  role of, 9–12
  social demands and, 222–224
  state government support of, 53, 59–60,
    222
  tenure of deans of, 75
  university's role in, 203–207
  within larger university family, 61
Access to care
  academic medical center and, 86–87
  price competition and, 221–222
Accreditation, 57–58, 110, 115, 151, 152,
  195
Aged, *see* Elderly
Alcoholism, 141, 142
Ambulatory care
  federal programs for, 118
  hospitals and, 56–57
  medical education and, 118, 133–134, 141,
    143, 144, 150
American Academy of General Practice,
  144
American Association for Labor
  Legislation, 19
American Cancer Society, 23, 113, 127, 197
American Heart Association, 113, 197
American Hospital Association, 7
American Medical Association (AMA), 6, 19
  accreditation and, 115, 195
  health manpower needs and, 29
  medical education and, 47, 119–120, 123,

M

Manpower, and public policy, 29–32
March of Dimes, 197
Marine Hospital Service, 17–18
Massachusetts, 18, 146
Massachusetts General Hospital, 50
Mayo Medical School, 243
Medicaid, 5, 58
  academic medical center and, 96, 175
  access to health services and, 87
  ambulatory care under, 143
  enactment of, 24, 28
  expenditures of elderly on health care
    and, 3–4
  federal funding of, 163, 181
  health care costs and, 36–37, 93, 98
  hospital income and, 72, 134, 167, 173,
    175, 180
  medical education costs and, 187
  primary care services and, 99
  public policy debate over, 33–37
  reimbursement experiments in, 92
Medical center, use of term, 44
Medical education, 109–157
  ambulatory care in, 118, 133–134, 141,
    143, 144, 150
  biomedical research and, 48–49, 110,
    126–133, 151–152, 229
  clinical framework used in, 140
  context and conduct of, 109–157
  continuing medical education (CME)
    programs in, 114–115
  costs per undergraduate student in, 52
  curriculum changes in, 122–126
  delivery of health services and, 84–86
  diverse programs in, 110, 114
  education responsibilities of schools in,
    109–115
  family medicine in, 144–146
  federal support for, 60, 116–119, 136, 167,
    180–182, 201
  fellowship programs in clinical
    subspecialties in, 113
  financing of, 165–173, 186–188
  Flexner Report and, 47–51, 110
  focal problems approach to, 150–151
  geriatrics in, 146–148
  as goal or by-product, 137–140
  graduate students in biomedical sciences
    in, 113–114

  health care system and, 3, 6, 7, 8
  health services delivery model in,
    231–234
  historical development of, 45–54, 110–111
  hospitals and, 133–135
  needs of students and faculty in, 138–139
  new model needed in, 229–234
  physician distribution and, 31–32
  physician supply and, 30–31, 118–119,
    135–137
  primary care in, 143–146
  principles in, 139–140
  psychosocial dimensions in, 235–236
  public needs and, 141–142
  public policy and, 41, 184–189
  racial minorities in, 121–122
  residency training programs and, 49–50,
    111–113
  social sciences research in, 132–133
  specialties in, 110–112, 124
  support for, 115–120
  systems approach to, 152–153
  task of, 228–229
  teaching hospital role in, 49–51
  types of students in, 120–122
  women in, 121
  see also Academic medical centers
Medical establishment, and health care
    system, 6–7
Medical practice plan, *see* Faculty practice
    plan
Medical Research Council (MRC), 130
Medical schools
  advisory board in, 208
  chief administrative officer (CAO) of
    university and, 203–204
  clinical department funding in, 207–208
  community-based, 67, 149–153
  department chairmen in, 213–214
  executive committees in, 209, 241
  expenditures of, 166, 168, 171
  finances of, 165–173, 186–188
  governance of, 207–209
  hospital financial arrangements with,
    167–168, 176, 178
  hospital relationships with, 61–66
  revenue sources for, 166, 167, 168,
    169–170
  tenure of deans of, 75
Medicare, 5, 39, 58, 219, 222
  academic medical centers and, 96, 175

University of Illinois College of Medicine, 149, 150
University of Michigan, Ann Arbor, 104
University of North Carolina, 112, 136
Urban Institute, 182

V

Veterans Administration, 7, 19, 21, 187
Vietnam War, 29

W

Wagner-Murray-Dingell Bill, 22, 34
Ways, Peter O., 150–151
Welfare programs, 20
Western Reserve School of Medicine, Cleveland, 124–125, 196
White House Conference on Health, 29
Wilson, M. P., 199, 213
Women, in medical education, 121
World War I, 19, 33
World War II, 20–21, 33, 34, 116

About the Authors

Irving J. Lewis is Professor of Public Policy and Community Health at Albert Einstein College of Medicine, Bronx, New York. In 1970 he concluded a long career in the federal government as Deputy Administrator of the Health Services and Mental Health Administration in the Department of Health, Education, and Welfare. Previously he had worked for many years in the Executive Office of the President, helping to shape the policies, plans, and budgets of a wide range of social and economic programs, both foreign and domestic. Professor Lewis has published extensively in professional journals and other publications. He frequently serves on health policy task forces, and was Staff Director of the Governor's Special Advisory Panel on Medical Malpractice in New York. He is a member of the Institute of Medicine of the National Academy of Sciences. He is a graduate of Harvard College (A.B.) and the University of Chicago (A.M.).

Cecil G. Sheps has been Vice Chancellor for Health Sciences at the University of North Carolina at Chapel Hill and is now Taylor Grandy Distinguished Professor of Social Medicine in its Medical School. During forty years of teaching, research, organizing, and administering health services, he has held significant positions in such institutions as the Beth Israel Hospitals of New York and Boston, Harvard University, the University of Pittsburgh, and Mount Sinai School of Medicine in New York. Dr. Sheps is a frequent consultant to institutions and governments in this country and abroad. He currently serves as a member of the Institute of Medicine of the National Academy of Sciences and of the Executive Board of the American Public Health Association. He received his M.D. from the University of Manitoba and his M.P.H. from Yale University. He has published over 120 articles in scientific journals and is the author or editor of eight books.